The
Overnight Diet

The Overnight Diet

Start losing weight tonight, and keep it off permanently

DR CAROLINE APOVIAN
WITH FRANCES SHARPE

Nutritional consultant Diana Cullum-Dugan RD
Exercise consultant Wayne Westcott Ph.D.

piatkus

PIATKUS
First published in the US in 2013 by Grand Central Life & Style
First published in Great Britain in 2013 by Piatkus

Copyright © 2013 Caroline Apovian and The Philip Lief Group Inc.
Developed by The Philip Lief Group Inc.

A CIP catalogue record for this book
is available from the British Library.

Note: The names of the individuals featured in the case studies
in this book have been changed.

ISBN 978-0-7499-5818-3

Illustrations by Joung Park
Designed and typeset in Calluna and Museo by Paul Saunders
Printed and bound in Great Britain by Clays Ltd, St Ives plc

Papers used by Piatkus are from well-managed forests
and other responsible sources.

MIX
Paper from
responsible sources
FSC® C104740

PIATKUS
An imprint of
Little, Brown Book Group
100 Victoria Embankment
London EC4Y 0DY

An Hachette UK Company
www.hachette.co.uk

www.piatkus.co.uk

To my mother, Ines Chinni Apovian,
who has always been ahead of her time.

About the Authors

Dr Caroline Apovian

During her time at university, Dr Caroline Apovian gained weight before developing the seeds of this plan to help her slim down and shape up. Based on her own success, she wanted to share what she had learned. Helping others safely achieve rapid weight loss that lasts became her life's mission. For over 25 years, Dr Apovian has held a position at the forefront of the obesity and weight-management field. One of the world's premier weight-loss experts, she has distinguished herself as a leading researcher, treatment provider and teacher in the fields of obesity and weight loss while also working as Director of the Nutrition and Weight Management Center at the Boston University Medical Center, Co-Director of the Nutrition and Metabolic Support Services at the Boston University Medical Center, Director of Clinical Research at the Obesity Research Center Boston University Medical Center, and Professor of Medicine at Boston University School of Medicine.

Her federal government positions include Nutrition Consultant to NASA, and appointed member of the federal government's panel on the evaluation and treatment of overweight adults.

Her unparalleled accomplishments in the obesity and weight-loss field, which have earned her recognition from her peers and made her a media favourite, include: her popular weight-loss column on EverydayHealth.com; recipient of the Physician Nutrition Specialist Award presented by the American Society of Clinical Nutrition for advancing nutrition education among doctors and medical students; grants from diverse sources, ranging from the National Institutes of Health and The Atkins Foundation to the Global Health Primary Care Initiative; and television appearances, from *The Dr Oz Show* to the Discovery Channel. She is also a frequent national and international lecturer.

Dr Apovian has published papers, reviews and book chapters on nutrition, obesity and nutrition support and serves as manuscript reviewer for several prestigious journals, including *New England Journal of Medicine, Journal of Women's Health, International Journal of Obesity, Obesity Research, Digestive and Liver Disease* and *Journal of Parenteral and Enteral Nutrition*.

Her editorial positions have included *International Journal of Food Safety, Nutrition and Public Health* (Associate Editor), *BMC Research Notes* (Associate Editor), *Current Opinion in Endocrinology and Diabetes* (Editor of the Nutrition and Obesity section), *Obesity* (Associate Editor), *Nutrition in Clinical Practice* (Associate Editor) and *American Journal of Clinical Nutrition* (Guest Science Editor). Her professional activities also include serving as: Chair of the Obesity Research Interest Section for the American Society for Nutrition; Principal Investigator for the Center for Obesity Research and Education; Executive Committee Member of the Boston Nutrition Obesity Research Center; Member of the Task Force on Physician Credentialing in the Obesity Medicine Subspecialty; Director of the Nutrition Support Fellowship; Director of the Nutrition and Obesity Medicine Fellowship; and Associate Director of the Graduate Program in Medical Nutrition Sciences.

Dr Caroline Apovian lives in Waban, MA with her husband and two sons. Her website is www.OvernightDiet.co.uk and her Facebook page is www.facebook/dr.caroline.apovian.

The Overnight Diet has been developed over many years and is the result of painstaking research. If you are interested in finding out more about the research used – and the research Dr Apovian has been involved in – you will find details on www.OvernightDiet.co.uk.

Diana Cullum-Dugan

Diana Cullum-Dugan, RD, LD RYT, is a licensed Dietician Nutritionist as well as a registered yoga teacher who began working with Dr Apovian in 1999. As a 'plump 12-year old with overweight aunts', Diana recognised a strong familial tendency to gain weight. To combat her predisposition, her parents sent her to a health spa, setting her on her career path of helping people interested in weight loss. At the Boston Medical Center, Diana managed the outpatient Nutrition and Weight Management Center and multiple clinical nutrition trials. At the same institution, she was the lead yoga teacher in a study for Yoga for Low Back Pain and is the exercise and nutrition expert on a respected web-based nutrition/exercise intervention programme.

Diana regularly lectures on weight management and nutritional assessment to wide audiences at Harvard University Medical School, Boston University's Sargent College, Northwest University School of Medicine and the American Dietetic Association.

Wayne L. Westcott

Wayne L. Westcott, Ph.D., directed fitness research programmes at the South Shore YMCA in Quincy, MA for more than 25 years. Wayne has been a strength-training consultant for numerous organisations, including the US Navy, the American Council on Exercise and the YMCA of the USA. He has authored or co-authored 24 books and textbooks and more than 60 peer-reviewed papers. Wayne serves as an editorial advisor, reviewer, writer or columnist for many publications, including *Prevention*, *Shape*, the *Physician and Sportsmedicine*, and ACSM's *Health & Fitness Journal*. He has been the keynote speaker for national meetings of the American College of Sports Medicine, the American College of Nutrition and the National Intramural and Recreational Sports Association. Wayne has served on the Executive Committee for the New England Chapter of the American College of Sports Medicine, as well as on the Advisory Boards for the International Council on Active Aging and for the International Association of Fitness Professionals. He has received the Lifetime Achievement Award from the International Association of Fitness Professionals, and the Healthy American Fitness Leader Award from the President's Council on Physical Fitness and Sports.

Frances Sharpe

Frances Sharpe is a writer and ghostwriter who has been covering health and wellness, fitness and diet for nearly 20 years. She is the ghostwriter of two *New York Times* bestsellers as well as 17 other well-received non-fiction books. Her work has also appeared in the *Huffington Post*, *AARP – The Magazine*, *Entrepreneur*, *Health*, *Women's Health & Fitness*, *Muscle & Body* magazine, *WellBella* magazine, *Teen People* and Playboy.com.

Important! If you have kidney disease or diabetes, check with your doctor before starting The Overnight Diet.

Contents

PART 4 The Overnight Diet for Life!

Acknowledgements

This book could not have been written without the help and dedication of a team of people around me sharing their expertise to create *The Overnight Diet*. Thank you to Frances Sharpe, and her ability to put it all together; to Diana Cullum-Dugan, whose creative ideas and recipes have no rival; to Wayne Westcott, whose enthusiasm for health and wellness is infectious; and to Rita LaRosa Loud, who makes it all happen in the fitness world. Thank you to photographer Thomas Huynh, who worked closely with Wayne Westcott and Rita LaRosa Loud to capture the fitness moves so eloquently. Thank you to illustrator Joung Park, who then transformed those photographs to the beautiful and simple, easy-to-follow illustrations you see in this book.

A big thank you to the team at Grand Central Publishing, especially Diana Baroni and Amanda Englander, both there 24/7 and ready to offer a solution for every little thing.

Also, thank you to Claudia Dyer and Jillian Stewart, for bringing my work to dieters in the UK and Australia.

Thank you to David Blackburn and Rod Egger, who invited The Overnight Diet programme into their realm because the philosophy was so closely aligned, and now we have the

Physicians Weight Loss Smoothie line. Thank you to George Blackburn, my mentor and now a dear friend, who always steered me the right way, and sees above everyone else.

And a special thank you to Philip Lief, the other person who also sees above everyone else!

Thank you to my father, Dr John Apovian, for believing in me, always. And last but not least, thank you to my little family, the Baker boys, Gus, John and Philip, for supporting me no matter what.

Introduction

Overnight results that last – that's what you get with the Overnight Diet. And it's a big part of how, in the past 20-plus years, I've helped my patients lose over 1 million pounds – that's over 71,000 stones or 453,500kg. You see, helping people to slim down is what I do. I'm not a cardiologist or a family doctor, or a hospital doctor who dabbles in weight management on the side. I'm an obesity medicine physician, which means that I specialise in weight loss. As the Director of the Nutrition and Weight Management Center at Boston Medical Center, I've helped thousands of people just like you to quickly and safely lose weight for good. And as one of the world's leading researchers on obesity and weight loss, I'm privy to – and sometimes I'm the one presenting – the most up-to-the-minute scientific findings on what makes people fat, what keeps them fat and what works to help them lose that fat for ever. In fact, my research colleagues have made a revolutionary scientific discovery that shows why most popular diets are doomed to fail. It's because they lead to muscle wasting – a condition known in medical circles as sarcopenia – that sabotages efforts to lose weight. We'll get to the details on that later. For now, just know that I am here to help translate this research and to use it to help you lose weight and keep it off.

The Dark Ages of dieting

Dieting has become stuck in the Dark Ages. I pay attention to every diet that comes out because my patients have usually tried them all and failed. It's no wonder. Most are either re-hashing the same advice or introducing wacky concepts that aren't based on any research at all. That's why, despite your best efforts, you haven't been able to lose that stubborn flab. Or maybe you have lost weight but can't seem to keep it from creeping back onto your thighs, bottom and belly, leading to a lifetime of yo-yo dieting. Or perhaps you're a few pounds or kilos lighter but still feel and look a bit flabby. Is that what you want after all that hard work – a jiggly midriff?

You probably feel frustrated and discouraged. I don't blame you. I've been there myself. I know from personal experience just how hard it can be to lose weight with most diets. When I was at university, I gained what is known in the US as the 'Freshman 10', then I went on to achieve the 'Sophomore 15' and the 'Junior 20' before slimming down and shaping up with what became the Overnight Diet. I listen with great empathy as my patients tell me all the reasons why they hadn't succeeded at dieting; for example, Tina, 27, lamented that one low-calorie diet left her feeling hungry all the time. Jenny, a 43-year-old mother of two, complained that she would lose a few pounds then see her weight loss come to a grinding halt even though she was practically starving herself. And 51-year-old Roger told me he would get beyond bored eating the same few bland foods on a diet's 'approved' list. The result? They all gave up and went right back to their old eating habits. They each told me that they felt like a failure. But I reassured each of them that they hadn't failed dieting; the Dark Ages diets had failed *them*.

It's bad enough when these diets can't help you reach your goal weight. But for some of my patients, trying to lose weight with popular diets has had far more dangerous consequences. I've had patients develop high blood pressure, high cholesterol, type-2 diabetes, gout, excruciatingly painful kidney stones or seen their muscles wither away – all from trying to lose weight and get healthy. It doesn't make any sense!

I have news for you. Losing weight shouldn't make you suffer. Slimming down – when you do it the right way with a bounty of nutritious foods – should enhance your health and well-being and make you feel better, not worse! Hearing what other diets were doing to my patients infuriated me. Seeing that so many of them were not losing weight with existing diet plans and that they were also harming their health, and feeling deprived and depressed, I knew I had to do something about it.

Developing the next generation of dieting

After witnessing the struggles of my patients, it became my mission to engineer a 21st-century science-based diet that would help you safely achieve rapid weight loss that lasts. The Overnight Diet is that plan: a revolutionary diet based on nearly 25 years of research as well as testing with thousands of people just like you. It takes dieting to a whole new level with real, road-tested benefits.

The Overnight Diet is very simple, but before I give you the details of the programme I want to let you know how I developed it. Here's why: your health and safety are of the utmost importance to me – and they should be to you too – so I want you to understand that this isn't a fad diet to lose a few pounds at the expense of your health. Instead, it's backed by decades of scientific research showing that in addition to producing quick results, it promotes better health and even longevity. That's right – it's your ticket to looking better, feeling better and living longer.

For years in my clinic and at the lab at the Nutrition and Weight Management Center at Boston Medical Center, I had been using two time-tested rapid weight-loss strategies with great success:

The first came from Doctors George Blackburn and Bruce Bistrian, the renowned creators of a highly respected and widely used medically supervised rapid weight-loss diet. After my residency, I took a two-year fellowship with these revered weight-loss pioneers and soaked up as much knowledge as I possibly could. Their diet was developed to be used in a highly monitored setting; that is, the hospital. As successful as it was, I knew that it could be more accessible and therefore effective for many more people. Over the years, I refined and improved their diet, taking it light years beyond what they had ever imagined. I have modified it so that it is easier to use and so that you can eat more food, which allows you to benefit from the lasting results you want with no doctor supervision necessary.

The second is based on a simple dietary habit that has been the subject of decades of research showing that it produces overnight weight loss and a health boost so powerful it increases longevity. It's something humans have been doing for thousands of years: taking a temporary break from solid food. In fact, scientific evidence shows that this is something our bodies are genetically programmed to do. But most people in the West no longer engage in this once-common practice, and research shows that because of this, our genetic programming has started working against us by piling more and more fat onto our bodies. It's hard to believe, but the weight-loss aspect of this practice has not been explored effectively – until now. I have given this long-standing approach a modern-day reinvention to maximise its flab-fighting ability in the minimum amount of time. The result? Losing more fat faster.

Both strategies had helped my patients knock off unwanted weight, but I knew they could do even more. One day, one of the staff members at my practice drove up in her new hybrid car, and she started raving about the incredible mileage it got from the combined battery and petrol engine. Right then, the wheels in my head started turning, and I had a light-bulb moment.

What if I combined these two separate strategies into one turbo-charged, high-performance diet?

I immediately went to work developing the optimal blend of the best of both plans so that they would work synergistically – fuelling each other in a similar way to a hybrid car's battery and petrol engine working together – to maximise results. I spent years testing and refining this combo diet with real-life people and found that it not only speeds weight loss but it also shatters the typical obstacles to long-term success, making it the ultimate plateau buster. Finally! The next generation of weight loss is here now. So say goodbye to the Dark Ages of dieting and say hello to the world's first-ever hybrid diet designed to produce overnight results that last.

Adding even more muscle to the Overnight Diet

The synergy that arises from two diet strategies working in tandem is only part of what makes the Overnight Diet so different from any other diet you've tried. Through research, I've also pinpointed the main culprit that thwarts efforts to fight fat, slows metabolism, leads to yo-yo dieting, and can devastate health. And contrary to popular belief, it has nothing to do with a lack of willpower.

It's muscle wasting, sarcopenia, but which I prefer to call 'Shrinking Muscle Syndrome'. It is the loss of muscle mass, strength and function that may occur naturally with age, but that may also occur as a dangerous side effect of, or be expedited by, most popular weight-loss methods. The nutritional make-up of many diets can cause the body to rob your muscles for energy, leaving you thinner, but weaker and flabbier. Losing muscle from these diets explains why even though your scales may show that 'magic number', you still can't fit into your skinny jeans and you don't want to wear a bikini because you look flabby and out of shape. But it gets even worse.

If you regain the weight you lost, as an alarming 95 per cent of people on Dark Ages diets do, according to statistics, you need to know that it typically comes back as fat rather than as muscle, so there's even more blubber than before. Losing and regaining weight over and over and over throughout your lifetime can be especially harmful. Eventually, a person can balloon up like the Michelin Man and not have enough muscle to support all that weight. Think of trying to hold up a watermelon with a couple of cocktail sticks – you get the idea. It's what scientists call sarcopenic obesity, or fat frail, and it's a scary condition that makes it difficult for people to stand up or even get out of a chair without assistance. Imagine needing help just to go to the toilet or answer your front door – that's how debilitating it can be.

If our diets and weight-loss methods don't change, in ten years many more people will be in wheelchairs than ever anticipated. Most people who are trying to lose weight have no clue that they could be in danger of developing Shrinking Muscle Syndrome, but I guarantee that they'll be hearing a lot more about this condition in the coming months and years.

Preventing Shrinking Muscle Syndrome is the ultimate key to rapid weight loss that lasts, and it's why I've engineered the Overnight Diet specifically to maintain lean muscle while eradicating flab. Don't worry, this doesn't mean you have to become a bodybuilder or turn into the Incredible Hulk – in fact, you don't even have to lift a single weight. What I'm talking about are long, lean, strong muscles that make you look toned and fit. Isn't that what we all want? Just imagine how great it will feel to wave goodbye to someone and not feel that embarrassing arm flab flapping in the breeze.

Look better, feel better, live longer

There's more good news: every aspect of the Overnight Diet is designed to promote health and well-being. And I'm not just talking about long-term health benefits that you won't notice until you're in your golden years. You'll be thrilled to know that eating the good-for-you foods on this diet can have effects that enhance your health now. Look at what can happen during the first week alone:

- **Immediately**: compared to eating a fatty breakfast, like greasy bacon or buttery croissants, eating a breakfast such as the ones recommended on the Overnight Diet provides a better boost in mental alertness, so no more need for that third cup of coffee to try to power through those morning meetings at work.

- **Within 90 minutes**: starting just 90 minutes after eating a breakfast similar to what you'll be eating on the Overnight Diet, rather than having a muffin, a scone or a doughnut, the levels of the hunger hormone ghrelin are reduced and remain lowered for three hours. That helps keep your stomach from rumbling.

- **After 24 hours**: you'll lose up to 2 pounds (900g) overnight as your body flushes out excess water weight, which reduces insulin levels, improves insulin sensitivity and minimises bloating. Plus, it activates the fat-incinerating process.

- **By Day 2**: eating adequate protein throughout the day, as you'll be doing on this diet, helps knock out those afternoon energy crashes, so that you can power through your day.

- **By Night 2**: eating plentiful amounts of what I call 'lean carbs' boosts serotonin production in the brain and can enhance your moods and promote better sleep. Imagine waking up raring to go. Plus, when you sleep better, it helps balance your appetite hormones to control hunger, as well as reducing stress, reducing cravings and boosting energy.

- **After 1 week**: you could lose up to 9 pounds (4kg) in one week. In addition, you'll experience reduced hunger, fewer cravings, better moods, higher energy levels, more restful sleep and enhanced mental alertness. Higher energy levels pump up your desire to get moving with physical activity, which boosts production of a metabolic enzyme called AMP-kinase. In turn, this enzyme gives your energy levels an added boost, and it increases production of a hormone called irisin that helps you burn more calories.

Is the Overnight Diet for me?

Whether you want to lose 5 pounds (2.25kg), 1 stone (6.3kg) or 3½ stone (22.7kg), this hybrid diet will help you do it quickly and safely without feeling deprived. Even if you just want to drop those few extra pounds you piled on over the Christmas period, you can do it by following this no-fuss plan. In fact, reaching your weight-loss goal has never been so easy. With the Overnight Diet, you can:

- Lose up to 2 pounds (900g) overnight and up to 9 pounds (4kg) in the first week, and every week thereafter, until you reach your goal weight
- Prevent weight-loss plateaus
- Burn more fat faster
- Eat more food while losing more weight
- Exercise less while burning more fat
- Stave off hunger pangs
- Enhance your health

I've seen it work for thousands of my patients, and I want to see it work for you too. That's why I'm sharing this programme with you in this book. I want you to be able to experience what it feels like to get the rapid results you're looking for and to feel good while you're doing it.

Let's get started!

PART 1

How the Overnight Diet Works

CHAPTER ONE

·····················

Overnight Results
that Last

With the Overnight Diet, you get the benefit of not just one, but two diet strategies blended into one hybrid plan. Together, they give you the quick results you want – losing up to 2 pounds (900g) overnight and up to 9 pounds (4kg) in the first week – as well as helping you keep the weight coming off and staying off so that you can finally enjoy a long-term relationship with that sleek new shape of yours. Scientific research shows how each piece of this combo diet primes the body to respond better to the other, creating the optimal physiological conditions for rapid weight loss that lasts.

Tales of the Measuring Tape

'A lot of diets promise fast weight loss, but I couldn't believe it when I lost 2 pounds [900g] after the very first day.'
Harriet, 32, lost 1 stone 4 pounds (8kg) and 3 inches (7.5cm) off her waist

THE OVERNIGHT DIET AT A GLANCE

**1-Day Power Up
(day 1)**

Jump-starts weight loss overnight, accelerates fat-burning, primes the body to respond optimally to the 6-Day Fuel Up

**6-Day Fuel Up
(days 2–7)**

Keeps the fat coming off, feeds the muscles with the optimal amount of protein, fuels the body with an endless array of great-tasting good-for-you foods for healthy weight loss without deprivation

Thanks to this synergy, the Overnight Diet safely delivers rapid weight loss, burns more fat, turns off your 'fat' genes, reduces water retention and bloating, staves off hunger pangs and prevents plateaus. And all of that adds up to enhanced motivation. Of course, it's pretty easy to stay motivated when the number on the scales keeps going down and your waistline keeps shrinking week after week.

How does this combo diet get you slim fast? It starts with the 1-Day Power Up, which is based on one of the time-tested rapid weight-loss strategies mentioned in the Introduction. It is a dietary habit that humans have been doing for thousands of years: taking a temporary break from solid food. This age-old practice has been re-engineered for the 21st century to jump-start fat burning and weight loss overnight, while reducing hunger. That's followed by the 6-Day Fuel Up, which builds on the 'protein-sparing modified fast' created by Doctors Blackburn and Bistrian. 'Protein sparing' means that it preserves lean muscle mass, which you'll learn much more about throughout this book. The 6-Day Fuel Up reformulates the protein-sparing modified fast to keep your body in fat-burning mode while allowing you to eat a bounty of tasty foods you love, including peanut butter, avocado and, yes, even potatoes. Then you start the seven-day cycle all over again, back at the 1-Day Power Up, which reboots your fat-burning engine and promotes overnight weight loss week in and week out. Just keep repeating these two parts of the plan until you reach your goal weight and your jeans zip up effortlessly – it's that simple.

This combination primes the body, creating a sort of 'metabolic marvel' that maximises weight loss. So, what happens inside the body when you alternate the 1-Day Power Up and the 6-Day Fuel Up?

Burn more fat faster

The Overnight Diet is formulated specifically to start incinerating fat faster than other diets. Most diets make you follow a lengthy initiation phase to stimulate weight loss. In today's 'I want it now' society, who has time to wait around? This plan is engineered to turn on the process almost immediately. Thanks to the 1-Day Power Up, your body will begin using fat as energy as soon as 24 hours after you start the diet.

In order to keep your body in fat-burning mode, you need to shift gears and follow with the 6-Day Fuel Up. If you don't make the switch, the fat-burning process is more likely to stall. Years of testing on thousands of patients has shown that alternating back and forth between these two phases is the secret to keeping the fat coming off.

We need fat-burning now more than ever. If you're reading this book, then you probably already know that the number of overweight people is spiralling. In the UK, an estimated 60 per cent of adults are overweight, while in the US two-thirds of adults are overweight.

How much fat is too much? That's a question patients at the Nutrition and Weight Management Center at Boston Medical Center ask all the time. And it's understandable why. With so many millions of people expanding into the overweight and obese categories, it seems like being overweight is the new normal. But, as your parents probably told you when you were a teenager, 'Just because everybody else is doing it doesn't mean you should.'

....

CASE STUDY *Lydia*

One of my patients, Lydia, admitted that it took her a while to realise she had a weight problem because everybody in her family was overweight and many of her friends were too. Even though Lydia was more than 2 stone (12.7kg) above a healthy weight, she thought she was at a normal weight because that's what was normal in her social circle. Then she saw the Body Mass Index (BMI) chart and realised her weight put her in the obese category.

....

For decades, scientists have been using BMI as an indicator of a person's body fat and to determine if a person is underweight, normal weight, overweight, obese or even morbidly obese. But because so many people think the same way Lydia did about being at a 'normal' weight, it's better to think of it as a 'healthy' weight. So forget normal, and get healthy.

With the BMI chart, it doesn't matter if you're the skinniest one in a big family; it's all about the numbers. BMI is calculated using a ratio of height to weight. You can use the BMI chart on page 19 to see how your weight measures up. Do note, however, that BMI does have some limitations, because it doesn't take into account a person's muscle mass; for example, an elite athlete who is very muscular and has low body fat may have a BMI that indicates overweight, when they clearly do not need to lose weight. At the other end of the spectrum, someone with a very slight build, low muscle mass and a spare tyre may have a BMI that indicates healthy weight or even underweight, but they would benefit from losing fat and toning up.

Losing weight by the numbers

So what's your number? Whether your BMI is in the healthy range and you just want to maintain your weight, or you want to lose the last 5 pounds (2.25kg), or if you have 10 pounds (4.5kg) to lose to get into the healthy range, or your BMI is over 30, this diet can work for you. About 450 patients come to the Nutrition and Weight Management Center each month, and they all have unique needs, just like you do. That's why this programme has been created so that it will work whether you want to lose a little or a lot. Just look at how it worked for Angie and her mum Christina. Both wanted to lose weight, but each of them had very different goals.

....

CASE STUDY *Angie and Christina*

Angie, 28, just wanted to drop about 10 pounds (4.5kg) fast so that she could fit into a slim-fitting dress for her ten-year school reunion, which was three weeks away. The dress had fitted her perfectly a couple of months earlier when she bought it, but after that, she had to travel to three week-long work conferences where fattening foods were served up buffet-style and the high-calorie cocktails were flowing. When she got back home and tried on her dress again, the zip got stuck halfway up.

Christina, 55, had been waging a war with fat for nearly 30 years and wanted to lose about 3 stone (19kg). She was very frustrated that she hadn't worked out a way to win the battle, even though she felt like she'd been dieting her entire life.

They both started the very next day on the 1-Day Power Up and followed it up with the 6-Day Fuel Up. Overnight, Angie lost 1 pound (450g) and Christina dropped 2 pounds (900g). By the end of the first week, Angie had lost 4 pounds (1.8kg) and Christina was 6 pounds (2.7kg) lighter. 'We were both amazed how much our bodies had changed in just one week,' Christina said. 'That was just what I needed to keep going.'

By the night of Angie's reunion, she had lost 11 pounds (5kg) and 2 inches (5cm) from her waist. 'My dress zipped up so easily,' she said. 'It actually felt a little loose at the waist. I could have worn a smaller size!' Her mum, Christina, stuck with the programme for six months and lost a total of 3 stone 5lb (21kg), 5 inches (13cm) off her middle, and 7 inches (18cm) off her hips. 'I don't think my body has ever looked this good,' she said at a follow-up appointment.

....

Get to know your fat cells

Many people think of the body's fat as the enemy, but your body needs fat cells to be healthy. Your body needs a place to store energy, and your fat cells do the job. Until recently, the theory was that we were all born with approximately the same number of fat cells – around 10 billion – and that number would grow until we reached adulthood, at which time the number of fat cells would remain the same. The belief was that if you consumed more calories than you expended, your fat cells would swell in size to accommodate that extra energy, but you wouldn't create any new fat cells. Based on this line of thinking, a lean person and someone who was 7 stone (44.5kg) overweight would have roughly the same number of fat cells, but the lean person's fat cells would be small and the overweight person's would be stretched like a balloon that's ready to pop. Now we know that it isn't quite so simple.

New research is revealing that the secret life of fat cells is far more complex. Overeating does cause fat cells to swell up in size, but when stretched to the limit, some of them may divide into two, and thus multiply in number, creating new fat cells. Theories now indicate that a lean adult might have about 10–20 billion fat cells, while an obese person might have as many as 100 billion.

Fat-burning – the basics

You know you want to burn fat, but how exactly does it happen? Getting that stubborn fat out of your body depends on a complicated bodily process, but to keep it simple, here are the highlights. The same way your computer needs a power supply to keep it running, your body needs energy for daily life. It's what allows you to walk from the car park to your office at work, play with your toddler or do housework. It's also required for a host of internal processes like breathing, keeping your heart beating, and thinking. You may be surprised to discover that this last one is quite the calorie burner – when you're at rest, your brain consumes about 20–25 per cent of your calories.

However, the body's number-one source of energy for all of these activities is glycogen, the form in which your body stores the carbohydrates you eat. The more daily activities performed, the more glycogen the body uses. If glycogen stores are completely depleted by these activities, then the body begins to burn fat as an alternate source of energy. When this happens, your body sends a signal to your fat cells to liberate their contents. The fat cells comply by releasing their 'stuffing' in the form of free fatty acids that enter the bloodstream – something called lipolysis. The fatty acids are then shuttled to the muscles, internal organs and other tissues, which burn it up for needed energy. This process is called oxidation. Once the fat is burned for energy, it's gone, and the fat cells that once housed it shrink. Skinnier fat cells translate into a skinnier you.

Body Mass Index table

Body weight (kgs)

Height (cms)	Normal							Overweight				Obese										Morbidly Obese														
BMI:	19	20	21	22	23	24	25	26	27	28	29	30	31	32	33	34	35	36	37	38	39	40	41	42	43	44	45	46	47	48	49	50	51	52	53	54
147	41	43	45	48	50	52	54	56	58	61	63	65	67	69	72	74	76	78	80	82	84	87	89	91	93	95	98	100	102	104	106	108	111	112	115	117
150	43	45	47	49	52	54	56	58	60	63	65	67	69	72	74	76	78	81	83	85	88	90	92	94	96	98	101	103	105	108	110	112	114	117	119	121
152	44	46	49	51	54	56	58	60	63	65	67	69	72	74	76	79	81	83	86	88	90	93	95	98	100	103	105	107	109	111	113	116	118	121	123	125
155	45	48	50	53	55	58	60	62	65	67	69	72	74	77	79	82	84	86	89	91	93	96	98	101	104	107	108	112	115	117	120	122	125	127	129	—
158	47	49	52	54	57	59	62	64	67	69	72	74	77	79	82	84	86	89	92	94	97	99	101	104	107	109	112	114	116	119	121	124	126	129	131	134
160	49	51	54	56	59	61	64	66	68	72	74	77	79	82	84	87	89	92	94	97	100	102	105	108	110	112	115	117	119	121	124	126	128	130	133	136
163	50	53	55	58	60	63	66	68	71	74	77	79	82	84	87	89	93	95	98	100	103	105	108	111	113	116	119	121	124	127	129	132	134	137	140	142
165	52	54	57	60	62	65	68	71	73	76	79	82	84	87	89	93	95	98	101	104	106	108	112	114	117	119	122	125	128	131	133	136	139	142	144	147
168	54	56	59	62	64	67	70	73	75	78	81	84	87	90	93	95	98	101	104	107	109	112	115	118	120	123	126	129	132	135	137	140	143	146	149	152
170	55	58	61	63	66	69	72	75	78	81	84	87	90	93	96	98	101	104	107	110	113	116	118	122	124	127	130	133	137	139	142	145	147	150	153	156
173	57	59	63	65	68	72	74	78	80	83	86	89	92	95	98	101	104	107	110	113	116	119	122	125	128	131	134	137	140	143	146	149	153	155	158	161
176	58	61	64	68	70	73	77	80	83	86	89	92	95	98	101	104	107	110	113	117	119	122	126	129	132	135	138	141	144	147	150	153	156	160	162	166
178	60	63	66	69	73	76	79	83	86	89	92	95	98	101	104	107	110	113	117	120	123	126	129	132	136	139	142	145	148	152	155	158	161	164	167	170
180	62	65	68	71	73	78	81	84	88	91	94	98	100	104	107	110	113	117	120	123	127	130	133	137	140	143	146	150	153	156	159	162	166	169	172	175
183	64	67	70	73	78	80	83	87	90	93	97	100	103	107	110	113	117	120	123	127	130	133	137	140	143	147	150	153	157	160	164	167	170	173	177	180
185	65	68	72	75	79	83	86	89	93	96	99	103	106	109	113	117	120	123	127	130	134	137	141	144	147	151	154	158	161	165	168	171	175	178	182	185
188	67	70	74	78	81	84	88	92	95	99	102	106	109	113	116	120	123	127	130	134	137	141	145	148	152	155	159	162	166	169	173	176	180	183	187	190
191	69	73	76	80	83	87	91	94	98	102	105	109	112	116	119	123	127	130	134	137	141	145	148	152	156	159	163	166	170	173	177	181	185	188	192	196
193	71	74	78	82	86	89	93	97	100	104	108	112	115	119	123	127	130	134	138	142	145	149	152	156	160	163	167	171	175	179	182	186	190	193	197	201

Turn off your 'fat genes'

Did you know that your genes may be working against you to make you fat? Genetic scientists have introduced the 'Thrifty Gene Hypothesis', which suggests that in prehistoric times certain genes helped our ancestors Caveman Joe and Cavewoman Jane thrive in times when food was scarce.

According to this theory, these genes played an important role in a natural cycle that alternated between feasting on food and then engaging in physical activity to hunt for their next meal. When Caveman Joe and Cavewoman Jane were successful at bringing home a wild animal for dinner, they would feast, and the so-called thrifty genes would go to work to store that food as fat. When the food supply ran out, Caveman Joe had to run, jump and climb to hunt down their next meal while Cavewoman Jane walked, squatted down and reached up high to gather plants and berries. That's when their fat stores would be burned as fuel. Feasting and storing fat; hunting and gathering for food and burning fat – that's the natural cycle our bodies were genetically programmed to follow and it's what kept Caveman Joe and Cavewoman Jane lean and athletic. (Have you ever seen a cave drawing of a fat caveman?)

Since those prehistoric times, our diets have changed dramatically. We now have an endless supply of food that we graze on constantly. And the only 'hunting' needed to acquire it is slowly strolling up and down the supermarket aisles. The nonstop eating and sedentary lifestyle means we no longer complete the natural eating cycle. Some scientists suggest that our diets have evolved but our genetic programming hasn't caught up, and those genes that proved to be such a lifesaver for our ancestors are now making us fat and unhealthy. These experts contend that we've become stuck in feasting mode, and our genes are simply doing their job by storing more and more fat on our bodies. Not only is this expanding our waistlines but it's also contributing to chronic diseases and poor health. Of course, in reality, it's far more complicated than this, but it is certainly possible that our genetics are working against us in the battle of the bulge.

The Overnight Diet is the antidote for this problem. It signals your genes to take a break from their job of storing fat so that your body can start burning it as fuel instead. Switching between the 1-Day Power Up and the 6-Day Fuel Up helps recreate the natural cycle our bodies were intended to follow so that we can get our genes working for us rather than against us.

Put your fat genes to sleep

Have you ever blamed your genes for your weight troubles? You could be right, at least partly. To date, scientists have identified dozens of fat genes. In fact, they discovered 18 new ones in 2010 alone, and some say there could be as many as 100 of them. But we don't all possess all of them. The discovery of fat genes helps explain why weight problems tend to run in families. A review of 46 studies involving nearly 124,000 people combined showed that the more fat genes a person has, the more likely they are to be obese. People with over 38 fat genes weighed an average of 15–20 pounds more than those who had fewer than 22 fat genes.

GET THE LOWDOWN ON THE SCIENCE

Were you born this way?

Scientists are beginning to find the answers to this question, and more are on the way. In 2011, the National Institutes of Health in the US gave a $2 million grant for a five-year study to investigate the impact of genetics on obesity and weight loss. Until the results of that study are revealed, here are

→

some of the existing findings on the role your parents might have played with regard to your weight:

- Numerous studies on twins show that being obese is 40–75 per cent hereditary.

- Researchers from London looked at 5,092 pairs of twins aged 8–11 and found that their BMI and waist circumference was 77 per cent hereditary.

- A study in the *Journal of Clinical Endocrinology & Metabolism* found that children born to a mother who had weight-loss surgery prior to pregnancy were less likely to be overweight than their siblings who were born before the mother had surgery. This suggests that a mother's weight during pregnancy may affect the developing foetus.

However, this does not mean that just because your parents were fat you are doomed to be fat too, or that there isn't anything you can do about it. Your genes are not your destiny! Your daily habits play a major role in what is called the 'expression' of those genes. This means that your behaviours can effectively turn on or turn off those genes. Having a muffin for breakfast and hitting the takeaway for greasy fast-food lunches and dinners every day can power up those genes to start fulfilling their mission of making you fat. But give your body the delicious healthy foods you will be eating on this diet, and it will help to put those fat genes into sleep mode.

Rev up metabolism

Metabolism is a complex bodily process that determines how quickly your body converts food into fuel and how fast it burns that fuel. It is part of the reason why some people can have a blowout at the all-you-can-eat buffet and still stay slim while the rest of us merely look on with envy. A sluggish metabolism is often blamed when diet after diet has failed.

Several factors play a role in determining the speed of your metabolism, including your age, gender and genes. After you hit the age of 40, your metabolism slows by about 5 per cent each decade. Women tend to burn fewer calories than men because they typically have less muscle mass than men. And those genes you inherited from mum and dad also count. But so does your body composition and your activity level. One of the main reasons your metabolism slows is that with age people tend to lose muscle mass through a process called sarcopenia, as mentioned earlier, but we'll get to that in Chapter 2.

Weight-loss doctors use a rather complicated equation to determine a person's resting basal metabolic rate (BMR). That's the number of calories your body uses just to perform all its basic functions, like breathing, digesting and keeping your blood circulating. There's no need to bore you with the maths here, but basically it means that a woman who is 5 foot 5 inches (1.65m) and weighs 14 stone (89kg) burns more calories on those basic functions than a woman who is the same height but weighs only 9 stone (57kg). Now let's say that a 14 stone (89kg) woman loses 3½ stone (22.7kg). This means her body now uses fewer calories on basic functions, so she needs to eat less to maintain her body weight.

When you carry extra weight, it causes your body to work harder to perform all the necessary processes of life. That's why, when you try a new diet that simply cuts calories, you probably lose weight easily at first, but then it gets harder and harder to keep it coming off. Your BMR naturally declines as you lose the weight. It simply doesn't have to work as hard to keep your body functioning. So even though you're consuming the same amount of calories on your diet, you may stop losing weight, which can make you want to quit your diet.

Tales of the Measuring Tape

'I always thought it was my metabolism that was preventing me from losing weight. A couple of my girlfriends and I tried a few diets together and they all lost weight easily (of course, they put it all back on!) but I would lose a few pounds then hit a plateau. I was ready to give up entirely and felt like I was destined to be fat for the rest of my life. Now I know why my metabolism was working against me. We were all eating the same number of calories per day, but because I weighed about 5 stone (31.75kg) less than they did to start with, I dropped fewer pounds. Plus, even though I stuck within the calorie restrictions, I was eating foods and doing exercises that did nothing to boost my metabolism. With the right foods and the easy workout on the Overnight Diet, I actually lost more weight than my girlfriends!'
Andrea, 29, lost 2 stone (12.7kg) and went down four sizes in trousers

That's part of the reason there is no calorie counting on the Overnight Diet. The synergy of this combo diet is designed to avoid this common problem and speed up your metabolism as you lose weight so that you can keep the weight coming off – even if you've got age, gender and genes stacked against you. The nutritional make-up of the diet has been formulated with this specific goal in mind. You'll be eating lots of great-tasting, metabolism-boosting foods that will help you burn more calories faster. Plus, in Chapter 2, you will discover many more ways the Overnight Diet will increase your metabolism.

MYTHBUSTERS

Myth Yo-yo dieting permanently slows your metabolism and makes it harder to burn calories.

Many people think that because they have repeatedly lost weight through dieting and then gained it all back, that their metabolism is ruined and that it will be for ever stuck in a low gear. Although it is true that some diets may temporarily wreak havoc with your metabolism, their effects don't last.

Several studies have been published that put this myth to rest. In one, Canadian researchers looked at 52 overweight women who had been yo-yo dieters for an average of 18 years. They calculated the women's resting metabolic rate, then compared that number with what their resting metabolic rate would normally be, based on their ages, heights and weights. In more than 92 per cent of the women, there was no difference.

This doesn't mean that 'weight cycling', as doctors refer to yo-yo dieting, is OK or healthy. In fact, it can have detrimental effects on your health. But the message here is that even if you have been a lifelong yo-yo dieter, you can still whip your metabolism back into shape by following the Overnight Diet.

Reduce bloating by enhancing insulin sensitivity

Did you know that having high levels of the hormone insulin can cause the body to retain extra water, which can make you feel bloated? The Overnight Diet is engineered to produce a dramatic reduction in the body's production of insulin. Lowering insulin levels flushes excess water out of the body to help get rid of that puffiness. Without that extra water weight, your body will become more defined as you lose weight. Who knows, you just might have a six-pack lying underneath.

You may be wondering if losing water weight is good for your health. The answer is yes, as long as you're flushing out excess water. We all need to be properly hydrated for optimal health, and this diet will provide you with adequate fluids. It's the excess fluid retention that gives you that bloated look and which stresses your body and health. Too much fluid in your system strains your body's vital organs by making them work harder. When you release those extra stores of water, your body works more efficiently and you shrink down in size more easily.

MYTHBUSTERS

Myth When you lose water weight you will regain it quickly.

This myth may be true with other diets on which you lose water weight during an initiation phase only to regain it because the post-initiation foods you're eating don't reduce insulin levels. The 1-Day Power Up sparks that initial water weight loss, and the 6-Day Fuel Up keeps it from coming back. Alternating back and forth between these two parts of the Overnight Diet enhances something called insulin sensitivity. This means that insulin is working effectively at its primary job of regulating blood sugar, which helps keep water from accumulating in your body to prevent unwanted bloating. The 1-Day Power Up dramatically reduces insulin production, which enhances insulin sensitivity, and the 6-Day Fuel Up maintains insulin sensitivity at a high level to keep you from regaining water weight.

Boost human growth hormone, your body's natural flab fighter

Human growth hormone (HGH) is one of the most important natural hormones in the human body. Produced by the pituitary gland in the brain, it is involved in a variety of essential bodily functions, including reducing body fat, protecting lean muscle mass and maintaining metabolic balance. The higher the levels of HGH, the better the body performs these duties. With age, levels of growth hormone dramatically decline and have been associated with weight gain, muscle loss, wrinkles, weakness and more. You may have heard of HGH before. Athletes, celebrities and people looking for the fountain of youth are reportedly taking it for performance enhancement, injury recovery, weight loss and anti-ageing. And supplement manufacturers are trying to cash in with products promising to stimulate HGH production.

Let's be perfectly clear here: the Overnight Diet does not suggest that you take HGH supplements to help you achieve your weight-loss goals.

However, the Overnight Diet will help boost HGH levels naturally. This diet, and the 1-Day Power Up in particular, has been engineered to kick HGH into high gear so that you can get slimmer faster. Researchers at the Intermountain Medical Center for Heart Health in Utah presented findings at the 2011 annual scientific sessions of the American College of Cardiology confirming earlier evidence showing that following a diet similar to the 1-Day Power Up for just 24 hours significantly accelerates production of HGH. How much? In women HGH levels jumped by an average of 1,300 per cent, and in men levels skyrocketed nearly 2,000 per cent. This doesn't mean that this diet is going to make you look 20 years younger overnight, but follow it to the letter and you will be leaner, feel more vibrant *and* look more youthful.

Prevent plateaus

Plateaus are one of the most common roadblocks to weight-loss success. For some people, it's their metabolism slowing down that causes the scales to get stuck. For others, it's sheer boredom eating the same few foods from a diet's 'approved' list that causes progress to stall. Whatever your reasons may be for hitting plateaus, this diet will make them a thing of the past. On the Overnight Diet, every seven days you can lose up to 2 pounds (900g) overnight with the 1-Day Power Up to shake up those plateaus week in and week out. Plateau problem solved!

....

CASE STUDY *Maria*

Maria, 31, had tried diet after diet but could never lose those last 5 pounds (2.25kg) to get to her goal weight. 'I thought I was going to be stuck with those stubborn pounds for ever,' she said. But switching from the 1-Day Power Up to the 6-Day Fuel Up did the trick. 'It worked,' she said. 'Finally reaching my goal weight after all this time feels so incredible. I look better than ever, and I feel better than ever too.'

....

Stave off hunger pangs

Is it really possible to lose weight and not feel hungry while doing it? Definitely! The Overnight Diet is specifically formulated to give you the results you want without the deprivation. This aspect is critical, because feeling deprived while dieting increases cravings and bingeing, which can sabotage weight-loss efforts. Thinking that you can never indulge in the foods you love most can also be downright depressing and demotivating. This plan was formulated with these issues in mind, which is why you won't go hungry, and you won't have to give up your favourite foods, such as bread, spaghetti and burgers.

The Overnight Diet emphasises nutrition that is high in lean protein and fibre, both of which have been shown to increase satiety. That means they help keep you feeling full longer, so your stomach doesn't start to rumble soon after meals. Plus, you'll have an all-you-can-eat option for fruit and non-starchy vegetables. There are no limits on these good-for-you foods, so you never have to go hungry while losing weight.

GET THE LOWDOWN ON THE SCIENCE

Satiety and the fullness factor

How do we know which foods provide the greatest level of satiety? One of the most interesting studies on foods and fullness comes from Suzanna Holt and fellow researchers at the University of Sydney. In an experiment, Holt and her team fed volunteers 38 foods to determine which types of food made them feel fullest the longest. According to their findings, foods with high amounts of fibre, protein, and/or water tend to be the most satisfying and are the best at preventing hunger. By contrast, foods that contain high amounts of sugar, fat and/or starch tend to provide less satiety and may lead to hunger pangs soon after eating.

Eat more foods, lose more weight

Most diets start with initiation phases that severely restrict what foods can be eaten; some turn antioxidant-rich fruit into a forbidden food, while others allow for little more than protein at first. But it's nearly impossible to stick with these types of diets. That's why this plan lets you enjoy so many of the foods you love right from the start. You won't have to cut out all carbs, forego dairy or cut fruit from your diet.

What will you be eating on the Overnight Diet? During the 1-Day Power Up, you'll be enjoying a unique blend of tasty, filling foods that you'll find in Chapter 3, and you'll learn all about the great foods you'll be eating on the 6-Day Fuel Up in Chapter 4. But just know this for now: from the very start, you'll be eating lean protein, low-fat dairy, healthy fats and 'lean carbs': whole grains, and all-you-can-eat fruit and non-starchy vegetables. There's also room in this diet for the things you really love, including dessert and wine.

The guidelines for eating are so simple with the Overnight Diet, you can forget about any arbitrary restrictions. Some diets tell you that the secret to weight loss is to stop eating carbs after a certain time of day, but there is no scientific basis for these claims! Rest assured, your body is just as capable of metabolising the calories from a slice of wholemeal bread or an orange at 8.00pm as it is at 11.00am.

Some diets claim that there are super weight-loss powers in specific foods and encourage you to focus on a particular food every single day, but these are just gimmicks. Scientific research shows us that there are hundreds of wonderful foods that can help you trim down, and you will find all of those foods in this book. Why force yourself to eat only a few of them? This diet gives you free rein to find the fat-busting, metabolism-boosting foods that you love. After all, you're more likely to stick with a plan that lets you eat the foods you enjoy than one that makes you eat the same thing day in and day out. With dishes like Beefy Mushroom Burgers, Rosemary Pork Roast, Diana's Magnificent Hearty Pancakes, and yummy desserts like Apple and Cranberry Crumble, eating healthily is a pleasure.

GET THE LOWDOWN ON THE SCIENCE

Say hello to lean carbs

Carbohydrates have received a bad rap in recent years, but the research shows that the low-carb craze got it wrong. Carbs are essential to a healthy diet and to losing weight and keeping it off. The Overnight Diet emphasises 'lean carbs'. These are whole grains, fruit and non-starchy vegetables, and they are a key component of this get-slim plan. A 2009 study in the *Journal of the American Dietetic Association* evaluated the diets of 4,451 adults and found that those consuming the most lean carbs were the least likely to be overweight or obese and those who ate the fewest lean carbs were the heaviest.

Enhance motivation

Nicole, 44, couldn't lose the 2½ stone (15.8kg) she'd gained since having her second child almost ten years earlier. She'd tried to diet and would lose some weight in the first few weeks, but then her motivation would wane and she'd give up. Nicole isn't alone. Nearly every patient at the Nutrition and Weight Management Center at Boston Medical Center has struggled with staying motivated while trying to lose weight. Most of them say that their enthusiasm starts to slip away when they hit one of those annoying plateaus or, even worse, gained a few pounds while dieting. And who can blame them? When the scales don't co-operate, you can feel like all your efforts are in vain.

With this diet, the weight will keep coming off each week, so it's easy to stay motivated. Just ask Nicole. After losing 2 stone 10 pounds (17.2kg) – three more pounds than her goal weight! – on the Overnight Diet, she said, 'Because I kept losing weight each week, it kept me motivated to keep going. That's never happened to me before.'

Success is a powerful motivator. And you'll probably feel that after just one day. When you wake up the morning after doing the 1-Day Power Up and you are already lighter, it will make you want to keep going. And when you see more weight come off with the 6-Day Fuel Up, it will only add to your confidence. Then you start over again with the 1-Day Power Up where you can lose up to another 2 pounds (900g). Having that powerful day in the plan is so important in retaining your motivation.

Achieve lifetime weight control

The Overnight Diet's combination of these two scientifically proven weight-loss methods will help you keep your weight under control for the rest of your life! This isn't a restrictive plan; the Overnight Diet is a way of life. The basic concept of alternating from the 1-Day Power Up to the 6-Day Fuel Up is something you can easily do for years to come and is the answer to keeping weight off for good.

. . . .

CASE STUDY *Annie*

Annie, 51, who lost over 2¾ stone (18kg) as a patient, has been following the Overnight Diet for four years now, and she says it's become second nature to her. 'I can't imagine eating any other way now,' she said. 'After reaching my goal weight, I made a few tweaks, but still follow the 1-Day/6-Day cycle. And now my husband does it too, even though he doesn't need to lose weight. We just love the way everything tastes and we like the way it makes us feel.'

. . . .

Like Annie, once you reach your goal weight, you too can make a few simple adjustments to the Overnight Diet to make it a plan for the rest of your life. (See Chapter 11 for details.)

Diet isn't the only factor in staying trim – and healthy – for life. Exercise is a vital component too. If exercise 'isn't your thing', don't worry, I'm not going to ask you to spend endless hours in the gym. The next chapter explains why exercise is so important – and why you don't need to do as much as you might imagine.

CHAPTER TWO

·····················

Adding More Muscle to the Overnight Diet

Taking two proven weight-loss methods – a temporary break from solid food and the protein-sparing modified fast – re-engineering them and combining them into one plan is only part of how this diet will turn your body into a powerful fat burner. There is another component that takes the synergy of this hybrid diet and makes it even more powerful: preserving lean muscle.

The amount of lean muscle in your body is one of the key elements in setting your body's metabolic rate and determining how quickly you use calories. The more lean muscle you have, the better your body is at burning fuel. The less you have, the slower your metabolism. The problem is that our diets and life-styles are robbing our bodies of the muscle that we need to help us incinerate fat and slim down.

Remember Shrinking Muscle Syndrome, which I talked about in the Introduction? It's the loss of lean muscle that occurs natu-rally as you get older. Starting at age 30, muscle mass begins to decrease by about 1 per cent each year. But it is also an unwel-come side effect of losing weight on many popular diets. On low-carb diets, you will lose some fat, but you will also lose some muscle mass. And what about those old-fashioned low-fat diets that are high in carbohydrates and low in protein? They can also rob the body of lean muscle.

Shrinking Muscle Syndrome is the giant pothole that sends you veering off the path to fast results and permanent weight loss, and derails your efforts for a slimmer, trimmer, healthier you. Let's explore how it causes fat-burning to sputter.

Shrinking Muscle Syndrome

When Shrinking Muscle Syndrome occurs, you may not even know it at first. But after some time, you may start to notice that walking seems to take a lot more effort than it used to. Climbing stairs may leave you huffing and puffing. But before you even notice these tell-tale external signs, a whole barrage of changes has already started taking place inside your body – changes that rob your body of muscle tissue and sabotage your ability to lose weight and burn fat.

Tales of the Measuring Tape

'I could barely get up the stairs to my bedroom without gasping for air, and I felt like I was dragging all the time. I thought that it was just because of all the extra weight I was carrying around. I had no idea that it was also due to the fact that my muscles were disappearing. When I learned about Shrinking Muscle Syndrome, it really made sense. Gaining muscle is what helped me lose the weight and get into the best shape of my life. Now I can run up the stairs!' Angela, 39, lost 6½ stone (41.7kg)

To help you understand the chaos that occurs inside your body, let's look at the major players in your muscle-building team and the changes that keep them from doing their job.

Mitochondria Inside your body's cells are mitochondria – tiny engines that take in nutrients and use them to provide energy. All of your cells have some mitochondria, but your muscles are absolutely packed with them, which gives your muscles the energy to walk, run, jump, push, pull, lift and so on. Your body is constantly regenerating mitochondria so that it can create the energy your muscles need to perform. But, as you age, this process slows down and two things happen: your body regenerates fewer mitochondria, and the mitochondria you do have become a bit sluggish. When your mitochondria no longer perform their job of converting nutrients into useable energy as efficiently as they used to, it results in less muscle tissue and slower response times from your muscles.

HGH In Chapter 1, you saw how HGH helps to fight flab naturally. HGH plays an essential role in cell development and regeneration, both of which are important for preserving lean muscle mass as you will learn later in this chapter. Higher levels of HGH have been associated with increases in lean muscle mass and reductions in body fat. As you age, the body's production of HGH slows to a crawl, and your muscles begin to shrink and weaken.

Insulin-like growth factor-1 (IGF-1) IGF-1 is a natural hormone that is produced in the liver that promotes cell growth and regeneration, particularly cells within the muscles. When levels of HGH rise, the liver pumps out more IGF-1, which has been associated with increases in lean muscle mass and decreases in body fat. Adequate levels of IGF-1 have been found to help in the prevention of the age-related degeneration of muscles.

When IGF-1 levels are insufficient, however, muscles tend to wither away and body fat increases. Low levels of IGF-1 can be caused by many factors, including nutritional deficiencies, such as those arising from extreme calorie cutting.

In essence, Shrinking Muscle Syndrome decreases your body's ability to perform muscle repair and to generate muscle tissue. It reduces the concentration of your body's natural fat-burning hormones, including HGH and IGF-1. Not only does your body generate less of these hormones, but it also responds more weakly to the hormones that are already circulating in the body.

Fat invades your muscles

Most people think that as we gain weight, the fat basically sits on top of our muscles, creating unsightly lumps and bulges under the skin. But we now know that isn't entirely true. New imaging studies reveal that as your BMI rises, fat infiltrates your muscles, further decreasing their ability to perform the most basic functions. Take a look at the illustrations below to see just how much fat invades the muscles as BMI increases. In these images, the dark areas are muscle, and the light areas are fat.

Fat Within Muscle Fibre at Different BMIs

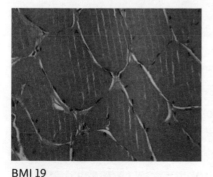 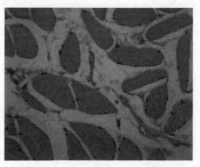

BMI 19   BMI 35

(Photos courtesy of Tom Storer, Ph.D., Boston University School of Medicine)

Once your body starts losing lean muscle mass and experiencing a decrease in the quality of the muscle fibre, it puts you on the motorway to Blubbershire. Weakened, withered muscles impair your ability to function, which makes you more likely to join the growing ranks of couch potatoes, and this in turn makes your muscles even weaker. It's another one of those vicious cycles that sabotage weight loss. What makes it even worse is that if you continue to eat the way you always have while these changes are taking place in your muscles, the weight starts to accumulate quickly.

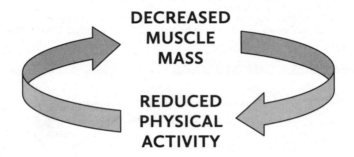

DECREASED MUSCLE MASS

REDUCED PHYSICAL ACTIVITY

Unfortunately packing on the weight is only the tip of the iceberg. Muscle loss can lead to a host of other metabolic problems that make losing weight nearly impossible. If the Overnight Diet works synergistically to create a sort of 'metabolic marvel' that helps you burn fat and lose weight, Shrinking Muscle Syndrome does just the opposite. It creates a metabolic mess that causes fat to stick stubbornly to your body.

In particular, Shrinking Muscle Syndrome is associated with insulin resistance, metabolic syndrome and inflammation – all conditions that detract from your body's ability to burn fat. Many of the patients at the Nutrition and Weight Management Center at Boston Medical Center have one or more of these problems, and what's really scary is that the vast majority of them don't even know it! It's like they have been waging a war against fat for years and years without realising that these chronic conditions are fighting against them. No wonder they have such a tough time losing weight.

Here's a quick look at how these conditions associated with Shrinking Muscle Syndrome sabotage weight loss.

Insulin resistance

When your body produces the hormone insulin but doesn't use it efficiently, this is known as insulin resistance. Insulin, which is produced by the pancreas, helps your body's cells use glucose for energy. Let's say you eat a burger, French fries and a shake at your favourite fast-food spot. Your body converts that food into glucose and your pancreas starts pumping out insulin so that you can use that glucose as energy.

With insulin resistance, however, your body doesn't use the hormone efficiently, so your pancreas keeps spewing out more and more insulin. As you remember, high levels of insulin can cause water retention. That's why insulin resistance is associated with carrying extra water weight, which makes you look and feel bloated. Insulin resistance also has a close relationship with fat and makes you more likely to be overweight or obese. It is linked especially closely to extra belly fat, which means that even if you lose weight on some other diets, you're likely to still be stuck with those love handles or a muffin top. Insulin resistance can also lead to excess amounts of glucose in the bloodstream and can set the stage for pre-diabetes or type-2 diabetes.

Tales of the Measuring Tape

'I didn't have a lot of weight to lose, but whenever I cut calories and lost a few pounds, I still felt bloated and could never get rid of that jiggly belly that would spill over the top of my jeans. I was shocked when my blood tests revealed that I had insulin resistance and was pre-diabetic! That was a big part of the problem and no amount of simple calorie cutting was going to fix that.' Sophie, 33, lost 12 pounds (5.4kg) and 2 inches (5cm) off her waist

So what does Shrinking Muscle Syndrome have to do with insulin resistance? Your muscles play a starring role in your body's ability to use insulin. The more lean muscle you have, the more effectively your body uses it. The muscle loss that occurs with age or from trying to lose weight with many popular diets reduces your body's ability to use insulin. The end result? More bloating, stubborn fat and, possibly, type-2 diabetes.

Once again, it's a double-edged sword. Muscle loss contributes to insulin resistance, and insulin resistance also promotes muscle wasting. It's like driving onto a roundabout and then picking up so much speed that you can't safely navigate to any of the exits. You get stuck going round and round and round. And once you get trapped in that loop, it's a speedy trip to another spare tyre around your middle.

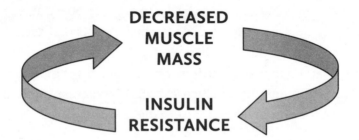

DECREASED MUSCLE MASS

INSULIN RESISTANCE

GET THE LOWDOWN ON THE SCIENCE

The Shrinking Muscle Syndrome–insulin resistance loop

In a 2010 issue of the journal *Plos One*, a team of scientists from UCLA analysed data from 14,528 people to see if muscle loss plays a role in insulin resistance. They found that muscle wasting was associated with insulin resistance not only in obese people but also in people who were not seriously

→

overweight. This means that even if you are losing weight on a diet, you could be setting the stage for insulin resistance if you are also losing lean muscle on that diet. And that will make it much harder for you to keep that weight off.

Metabolic syndrome

Metabolic syndrome is a cluster of conditions that increase your risk of heart disease, stroke and diabetes. The conditions associated with metabolic syndrome include the following:

High waist measurement Having too much blubber on your belly, or having an 'apple' shape, is a greater health risk than if you have a 'pear' shape. The following waist measurements are associated with metabolic syndrome:

Waist Size

Women	35in (89cm) or higher
Men	40in (102cm) or higher

High triglycerides Triglycerides are a type of fat in the blood. Having high levels of this type of fat increases your risk of the disease.

Triglycerides

Optimal	1.7mmol/l or less
High	1.77mmol/l or higher

Low HDL cholesterol HDL is often referred to as the 'good' cholesterol. Its primary job is to sweep cholesterol out of your arteries so that blood can flow freely. When HDL levels are low, there is a greater chance of cholesterol building up in the arteries and potentially creating a blockage or causing heart disease.

HDL Levels

	Women	Men
Optimal	1.5mmol/l and above	1.5mmol/l and above
Low	Less than 1.29mmol/l	Less than 1.03mmol/l

High fasting blood sugar Having a high fasting blood sugar level is an indicator of pre-diabetes or diabetes and is associated with an increased risk of serious disease.

Fasting Blood Sugar

Optimal	Below 5.5mmol/l
High	5.5mmol/l or higher

High blood pressure Your blood pressure measures the force of the blood as it pumps through your arteries. High blood pressure means your body is pumping blood with greater force. This condition is associated with a higher likelihood of heart disease and stroke.

Blood Pressure

Optimal	Below 120/80
High	130/85 or higher

Having any one of these conditions alone puts you at increased risk of disease, but that doesn't mean you have metabolic syndrome. Having all of these conditions together is what really ratchets up the health risk and makes it almost impossible for you to lose weight and keep it off.

Being overweight, and in particular having a large belly, has long been associated with metabolic syndrome, but guess what? Scientists have found that low muscle mass and decreased strength are also important risk factors for metabolic syndrome. This means that Shrinking Muscle Syndrome can put you on the road to this dangerous condition. So can losing weight – and muscle – on some other diets.

Inflammation

Inflammation is the body's natural response when we are exposed to foreign invaders, such as a splinter, a virus, bacteria or toxins. We need it on a short-term basis to fight disease and infection. But inflammation can become chronic, and this has been associated with heart disease, obesity, diabetes, Alzheimer's disease and more.

Scientists are just beginning to understand the link between fat, inflammation and muscle wasting; for example, scientific evidence suggests that fat tissue, especially abdominal fat, produces chemicals that promote inflammation. And emerging research is finding that chronic inflammation also accelerates muscle wasting. In the *Journal of Applied Physiology*, a study from Italian researchers examined the link between obesity, muscle strength and inflammation in 378 men and 493 women. The scientists looked at the waist measurements of the participants, tested their strength using a handgrip device, and checked their blood levels for inflammation markers. The results showed that the people with higher waist measurements and lower strength also had higher levels of inflammation. The researchers concluded that abdominal fat directly affects inflammation, which in turn negatively affects muscle strength.

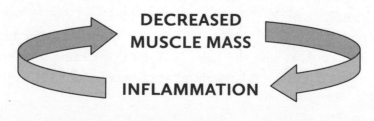

DECREASED MUSCLE MASS

INFLAMMATION

Common causes of Shrinking Muscle Syndrome

What shifts your body into Shrinking Muscle Syndrome gear? Of course, age has a hand in muscle wasting, but that's not all. Your diet could be putting you in danger of this condition. It may surprise you that a low-carb diet could pose a problem with muscle loss, but I'll tell you how it could happen. In addition, a lack of physical activity, and in particular a lack of strength training, can rob your body of muscle tissue.

The diet–Shrinking Muscle Syndrome connection

If you're like most people who are trying to lose weight, you may think you're doing your body a favour by following a typical low-calorie, low-fat or low-carb diet. But some of the most popular diet plans will ultimately fail to give you the sleek body you want and will leave your body feeling flabby instead of fit: research from my mentors Doctors Blackburn and Bistrian found that low protein consumption is also associated with muscle loss.

Many low-fat diets are also low in protein and high in carbo-hydrates. Many low-calorie diets offer no recommendations on daily protein intake, so you may not be getting enough of it to stave off muscle loss. And those low-carb diets? If you're cutting out healthy, whole-grain carbs while eating limitless amounts of fat and not consciously eating an adequate amount of protein, it could take a toll on your muscle mass. Not eating enough pro-tein can derail your dieting efforts because it sets the stage for Shrinking Muscle Syndrome and all the problems that come with it that make it so hard to lose weight and burn fat.

Thousands of the patients at the Nutrition and Weight Man-agement Center at Boston Medical Center have tried other diets but still couldn't lose the flab. They have the same problem: not enough protein! A large number of people fail to meet the official recommended intake. In the US, nearly 40 per cent of adult men and women eat less protein than the Recommended Dietary Allowance (RDA) of a minimum of 0.8g per 1kg of ideal body weight per day. In the UK, the so-called Guideline Daily Amount (GDA) for protein is 45g for women and 55g for men, while in Australia and New Zealand the Recommended Dietary Intake (RDI) is 46g for women and 64g for men. As you will see below, the Overnight Diet recommends more.

Tales of the Measuring Tape

'I was on one of those low-fat, low-protein, high-carb diets and couldn't work out why I wasn't reaching my goal weight. I was doing everything it said to do. When I told Dr Apovian what I was eating, she informed me that I wasn't getting enough protein. When I started eating the right amount of protein, I started losing weight fast – and I didn't feel starving any more!' Jamie, 27, lost 1 stone (6.3kg)

So what does protein intake have to do with maintaining lean muscle mass? A lot! Protein is the building block for your body's muscles. And every day of your life your muscles are going through a never-ending cycle of breaking down the proteins within and regenerating new proteins to replace them. To create these new proteins, your muscles need amino acids. Your body makes some of these amino acids on its own, but nine of them can be derived only from the foods you eat. These nine are called 'essential amino acids'.

Animal protein (meat, poultry, fish, seafood, eggs and milk) and soya foods contain all nine of the essential amino acids that your muscles need for rebuilding. When you don't eat enough protein, your body doesn't get the amino acids it needs to regenerate new proteins and it will continue breaking down your muscle, which ultimately leads to muscle wasting. Unlike carbohydrates and fat, the human body does not store amino acids for later use. This means that amino acids – in the form of protein – must be consumed every day in order to maintain muscle mass. Even one day of eating inadequate amounts of protein kick-starts the muscle-wasting process.

Inadequate protein intake = getting stuck in muscle breakdown mode

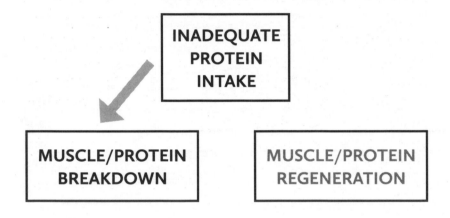

What's exercise got to do with Shrinking Muscle Syndrome?

Remember the Thrifty Gene Hypothesis? It is the theory that your genetic programming says your body is designed to follow a pattern of feasting on food and then hunting and gathering for your next meal. The 1-Day Power Up and 6-Day Fuel Up have been engineered to help recreate that natural cycle, but there's one more piece that fits into that cycle: physical activity. After all, when you have to hunt for your food, you have to run, jump and maybe even climb a tree. And gathering requires you to walk, bend, squat and stretch. And then if you're successful, you have to haul your dinner back home. That's a lot of work!

Here's how hunting and gathering works in today's society: some of us sit on the sofa and use our mobile phone or computer to order a takeaway. Twenty minutes later, the doorbell rings, and we get off the sofa to answer the door, then 'haul' the food back to the sofa to eat it. Successful hunting and gathering! Some of us grab our keys, drive to the nearest fast-food outlet, order (sometimes from a drive-through), and eat right there in our cars. Successful hunting and gathering! Some of us drive to the supermarket, shuffle up and down the aisles, fill our trolley with our favourite foods, then drive back home, pop something in the microwave and tuck in. Successful hunting and gathering!

Aside from the fact that it's a piece of cake to hunt down food in the modern world, the kind of foods we 'hunt and gather' are making it much harder to stop eating. We tend to gather and eat too much sugar and fat, which seems to produce inflammation throughout the body and even in the brain. In particular, inflammation seems to affect a region of the brain called the hypothalamus, which is the appetite and satiety centre. With inflammation here, your satiety mechanism goes haywire and stops sending you the signals that tell you you're full, so you keep eating and eating and eating.

Hunting and gathering in today's world is akin to shooting fish in a barrel: it's far too easy and requires barely any physical effort. The same effect can be seen in the rest of the tasks in our daily lives. Our society's focus on convenience has effectively turned us into sedentary beings and that's stripping our bodies of muscle. Scientists have shown that a sedentary lifestyle accelerates muscle wasting.

Being inactive isn't the only way to make your muscles wither away. Did you know that the exercise recommendations of many popular diets could actually be preventing you from reaching your weight-loss goals? And even worse, could be putting you in danger of muscle wasting? For decades, diets have been promoting aerobic exercise as the best way to burn calories and shed pounds. But the combination of very low-calorie diets with hours of cardio may be a recipe for Shrinking Muscle Syndrome, because it can put the body into a catabolic state in which it robs the muscles for fuel. During aerobic exercise, muscle proteins are broken down for energy. Adequate nutrition, and in particular protein, is necessary to regenerate those muscle proteins. If you don't consume adequate amounts of nutrients, especially protein, the muscles will begin to wither.

The Overnight Diet: the solution to Shrinking Muscle Syndrome

The Overnight Diet has been designed specifically to preserve lean muscle mass so that you can avoid Shrinking Muscle Syndrome and finally reach your weight-loss goals. It starts with getting adequate protein. What's adequate?

As I pointed out previously, it's more than current government recommendations. This conclusion is based on the research of Doctors Blackburn and Bistrian, pioneers in the field of nutrition and metabolism, as well as my own research and experience with thousands of weight-loss patients, which shows that a higher intake is needed to optimise weight loss and build up metabolism. To fuel fat-burning, you need to consume a minimum of 1.5g of protein per 1kg of ideal body weight. This is called your Daily Protein Requirement, or DPR as we will refer to it, and it's a critical component of this diet.

Let's say that your ideal body weight is 9 stone 4lb (59kg). At that weight, the US RDA indicates you should be eating approximately 47g of protein per day (in the UK the corresponding figure would be 45g for women, 55g for men, irrespective of weight). According to the RDA that 47g can come from any protein source, such as meat, fish, poultry, dairy, beans or high-protein vegetables. But experience and research show that this isn't enough to prevent muscle loss. On the Overnight Diet, you would be eating a minimum of about 89g of protein per day, and those 89g would come solely from lean beef, pork and chicken; fish; eggs; soya products; meat alternatives and protein powder. The protein found in other foods, such as dairy and beans, does not count towards your DPR, and there is no need to keep track of the protein in these foods. This will be explained more fully later.

What does that look like on your plate? You'll get the specifics in the coming chapters, but just to give you an idea for now: a breakfast that includes an egg and spinach omelette, a 140g grilled chicken breast wrap for lunch, and a 140g grilled salmon fillet for dinner would fill your protein needs. Of course, you would be rounding up those meals with other healthy foods.

Knowing your individual DPR is essential for success on this programme. You can use the Find Your DPR charts in Chapter 4 to help you determine yours.

GET THE LOWDOWN ON THE SCIENCE

The Power of Protein

In a seminal scientific paper published in the *Journal of the American Medical Association* in 1978, Dr Blackburn described the safety and efficacy of a protein-sparing modified fast: a low-calorie diet that included 1.5g of protein per 1kg of ideal body weight per day.

In a follow-up study published in the *Journal of Clinical Investigation* in 1984, Doctors Blackburn, Bistrian and colleagues compared the effects of a very low-calorie diet on nitrogen balance with either 0.8g or 1.5g of protein per 1kg of ideal body weight per day. Eating 0.8g of protein per 1kg of ideal body weight per day disrupted the dieters' nitrogen balance, but consuming 1.5g of protein per 1kg of ideal

→

body weight per day resulted in optimal nitrogen balance. Nitrogen is a compound that is used to measure a person's level of amino acids. When nitrogen balance is optimal, it means that a person has an adequate level of amino acids in the body for proper muscle regeneration. When nitrogen balance is skewed, it typically means that there are not enough amino acids in the body to halt muscle breakdown.

Research on protein consumption and the maintenance of lean muscle has continued since Dr Blackburn's first paper on the topic. A 2011 study from the University of Illinois shows that eating protein throughout the day is key to losing weight without sacrificing muscle. The study followed the dieting efforts of 31 postmenopausal women, all of whom ate a 1,400-calorie diet for six months. The women were divided into two groups, one of which received a powdered whey protein supplement twice a day and one that received a placebo containing an equal number of calories in carbohydrates. By the end of the study, the women who had consumed the additional protein had lost 3.9 per cent more weight and had a relative gain of 5.8 per cent more thigh muscle volume than women who didn't eat as much protein.

With an adequate amount of protein in your diet, your body will replenish the amino acids needed to halt the breakdown of your muscles and rebuild them. And by harnessing the power of protein to preserve lean muscle mass, you will be pushing fat burning into overdrive.

Pump up your muscles to power up fat burning

Because maintaining and adding lean muscle mass is the key to rapid weight loss that lasts, you won't have to dedicate big chunks of your day to aerobics in order to burn fat on this plan. Instead, you will be focusing on getting lean muscles through strength training. But don't worry. This is no run-of-the-mill weight-lifting routine. The same way this plan combines two diets into one for maximum results, it also integrates two exercise concepts into one to create a dynamic fat-burning session that lets you quickly strengthen and re-sculpt your body without ever having to lift a weight or spend hours on the treadmill.

Tales of the Measuring Tape

'You mean I can develop lean muscles and burn more fat without going to the gym or lifting heavy weights? Thank you!' Amanda, 44, lost 1 stone 5lb (8.6kg)

This unique workout plan relies on a growing body of research showing that combining resistance training with short cardio bursts (called 'Rev Up Blasts' here) into one workout burns far more body fat compared to doing strength training and cardio separately; for example, a pair of recent studies in the *Journal of Strength and Conditioning Research* compared the fat-burning effects of two types of workout routines. The first was a standard routine, including a weight-training session followed by an aerobic workout. The second was an integrated workout, in which people alternated weight-training exercises with high-intensity sprints. The combo workout outpaced the traditional routine in every area, including endurance, muscle strength and flexibility. But, most excitingly, the people who did the hybrid workout lost almost ten times more body fat compared to those who did the traditional workout.

The fun, fast-paced Quickie Rev Up takes only 21 minutes four times a week, requires no equipment, and can be tailored for all fitness levels, whether you're a workout newbie or a long-time exerciser. The easy-to-follow moves strengthen nearly every major muscle group in the body while improving balance and flexibility at the same time. And they are designed to help you move better so that you can do all the things you want to do, like playing games with your kids, taking your dog for a brisk walk, or going dancing with your spouse. It's fun, it's fast and it's functional for everyday life.

Building lean muscle with this strength-training programme will fuel fat burning by boosting your metabolism and by helping you avoid the conditions that keep you fat, including insulin resistance and metabolic syndrome. You have seen how Shrinking Muscle Syndrome increases your risk of these conditions. New research is showing that when you add lean muscle to your body, you can prevent or even reverse these conditions.

Several studies have shown that having low muscle mass is a risk factor for insulin resistance. But until 2011, no scientific research had attempted to find out if increasing muscle mass could reduce that risk. That's when a pair of researchers from UCLA analysed data from 13,644 people to test this concept. In their study, which appeared in a 2011 issue of the *Journal of Clinical Endocrinology & Metabolism*, they found that for every 10 per cent increase in muscle mass there was an 11 per cent reduction in the incidence of insulin resistance.

In the journal *Metabolism*, Australian researchers looked at a wide range of factors – age, muscle strength, muscle mass, hormone levels, medical conditions and marital status – and their association with metabolic syndrome. They found that muscle mass and strength were strong protective factors against metabolic syndrome. Their research also suggested that a substantial proportion of metabolic syndrome cases could be prevented with a strength-training programme.

A study from a Finnish researcher published in a 2011 issue of *Advances in Preventive Medicine* gets more specific about the benefits of strength training. It notes that resistance training has a favourable effect on metabolic syndrome because it decreases abdominal fat, enhances insulin sensitivity, improves glucose tolerance and reduces blood pressure values. The researcher concludes, 'Resistance training is probably the most effective measure to prevent and treat sarcopenia.' Because the Quickie Rev Up incorporates a form of resistance training, it will help you develop the lean muscle that fights Shrinking Muscle Syndrome and the conditions associated with it.

How to use this book

In the remainder of this book you'll find everything you need to incorporate the Overnight Diet into your daily life. Part 2 lays out the basic guidelines of the programme and shows you how to find your DPR, which is a critical component of this plan. In Part 3, you'll find dozens of quick-fix recipes and a 28-day meal plan to help you get started. Part 4 reveals the secrets to sticking to the diet wherever life takes you: on holiday, out with friends or grabbing food on the go. And in the final chapter, you'll discover how to modify the diet after you've reached your goal weight so that you can maintain your weight loss for good.

On the following two pages you'll find some fascinating information on why many typical diets are detrimental to health – and how The Overnight Diet differs.

Unfortunate dangers of typical diets

Early Death	Heart Disease	Type-2 Diabetes	Cancer	Kidney Problems	Moodiness/ Depression	Malnutrition	Constipation	Bad Breath	'Diet Flu'
A 2010 study found that a low-carb diet rich in animal foods was associated with a 23 per cent increase in mortality from all causes	Some low-carb diets with high-fat content and a lack of dietary fibre contribute to cardiac risk factors, including high cholesterol	The muscle loss that can occur with popular diets contributes to insulin resistance, which is a precursor to diabetes	Low-fibre, high-fat and low-carb diets may raise the risk of cancer	Diets that tell you to eat only protein for any amount of time have been linked to kidney stones and other kidney problems	Very low-calorie diets can make you feel lightheaded, mentally foggy and anxious. Low-carb diets can reduce serotonin levels, which can lead to blue moods	Diets that encourage you to cut back on entire food groups or even limit variety can lead to deficiencies in vitamins, minerals and other micro-nutrients	Constipation is a common complaint among dieters following low-carb eating plans and can be directly attributed to a lack of fibre in the diet	Low-carb diets and no-carb diets can cause embarrassing bad breath	Severe carbohydrate restriction causes withdrawal symptoms that mimic the flu, including headache, nausea, fatigue and an inability to concentrate

... and the Overnight Diet solution

Early Death	Heart Disease	Type-2 Diabetes	Cancer	Kidney Problems	Moodiness/Depression	Malnutrition	Constipation	Bad Breath	'Diet Flu'
Research shows that periodically enjoying a day like the 1-Day Power Up promotes a longer life-span. Studies show that a high-protein diet rich in vegetables similar to the 6-Day Fuel Up is associated with a 20 per cent reduced risk of death from all causes	By focusing on lean carbs that are high in fibre, the Overnight Diet helps protect your heart. 2007 research shows that routinely following a day like the 1-Day Power Up accounted for a 40 per cent reduced risk for heart disease	The synergy created by the Overnight Diet is the ideal recipe for reducing your risk for developing type-2 diabetes, and it could be your ticket to reversing the disease	This diet is overflowing with high-fibre, high-antioxidant, cancer-fighting foods. Research shows that high-fibre diets reduce the risk for colorectal cancer and that eating more fruits and vegetables reduces the risk of all types of cancer	This diet is high in protein, but it is also high in fibre, which helps kidneys flush protein out of the body and maintain optimal function	Abundant food on this diet prevents hunger, which cuts out the anxious feelings, light-headedness and mental fog. Lean carbs encourage serotonin production, which is associated with more stable moods	A wide variety of nutrient-dense foods from all food groups prevents any nutritional deficiencies	High-fibre foods will keep your digestive tract moving smoothly	Eating good-for-you lean carbs promotes weight loss and naturally fresh breath	Whole grains and unlimited fruits and non-starchy vegetables help make you feel great right from the start

PART 2

....

The Overnight Diet in Action

CHAPTER THREE

....

1-Day Power Up

On the 1-Day Power Up, you'll be enjoying a day of feasting on refreshing and invigorating jumbo smoothies – Banana Latte, Piña Colada Island or Enchanted Blueberry anyone? And you'll be doing this on a weekly basis until you reach your goal weight. There is one important caveat: as powerful and beneficial as the 1-Day Power Up is, don't do it more than once a week. Years of development and testing on thousands of patients have shown that once a week provides the optimal conditions to maximise its effectiveness.

The 1-Day Power Up was developed after patients at the Nutrition and Weight Management Center at Boston Medical Center kept complaining that they couldn't make it through those long, drawn-out initiation phases on other diets that required them to stick to short lists of approved foods for weeks or even months. 'Isn't there a faster way to lose weight?' asked Amy, a 27-year-old freelance graphic designer who had just got divorced and wanted to lose 1 stone (6.3kg) before jumping back into the dating pool. Amy grumbled that she could never make it through those ultra-restrictive start-up periods and always ended up giving up too soon. Amy's story is common. Perhaps you've caught yourself saying the same thing too.

Decades of research show that taking a periodic break from solid food can safely produce the rapid weight loss Amy and other patients were looking for. This was the inspiration to enlist the help of lead nutritionist Diana Cullum-Dugan to create something so delicious that people would actually look forward to it. The 1-Day Power Up isn't a day of deprivation, but rather a different kind of feast day. Twenty-five years of experience and knowledge about rapid weight loss, optimal nutrition and muscle maintenance went into the development of a menu of rich, creamy smoothies packed with protein, fibre and nutrients – not to mention lip-smacking ingredients like chocolate syrup, strawberries and yogurt.

Would patients like Amy like them? Would they be able to get through the whole day without feeling hungry or giving up? The science showed that metabolically, when combined with the 6-Day Fuel Up, it could do exactly what my patients were asking for, but how would it work in real life? The 1-Day Power Up smoothies were put to the test, and the patients couldn't stop raving about them. Amy told me she didn't feel hungry, and when she combined it with the 6-Day Fuel Up, she lost the 1 stone (6.3kg) fast enough to feel confident about dating again. She loved it. And you will too.

At first, the idea of a smoothie feast day once a week may seem a bit drastic to you. That's understandable. After all, our society, the food industry and many diet books force-feed us on the notion that we should be grazing constantly throughout the day. Rest assured that humans have been regularly taking breaks from solid food for thousands of years. Consider that even today, almost every major religion encourages this practice at certain times of the week, month or year. Millions of people take a break from their usual fare for specific periods of time for religious or other reasons. Did you know that Michelle Obama routinely enjoys a modified two-day food break? That's right. The First Lady, who has made it her mission to fight obesity in America, told *Ladies Home Journal* that she likes to take a periodic break from her regular meals to cleanse her palate and reduce cravings. And of course, remember Caveman Joe and Cavewoman Jane who thrived even when they were looking for their next meal.

The human body is designed to work extremely efficiently during this period. It's when the body taps into its stores and burns them for fuel. Each and every one of us already engages in this practice on a daily basis – it's just that we typically do it at night while we're sleeping.

Besides, with three jumbo smoothies that include real foods, this is not your typical 'juice day'. It's a veritable feast with a wide variety of rich, tasty drinks, including sweet smoothies, like Orange Zest, Chocolate Banana Swirl and Tropical Medley; savoury smoothies, like Kale Margarita; and veggie-packed 'green' smoothies, like Green Machine. Some of them are so big, you probably won't be able to finish them in one sitting, which means you'll have enough leftover for a tasty snack later in the day. And when you wake up the next morning and hop on those scales, you'll be amazed how easy weight loss can be.

Get-started guidelines for your 1-Day Power Up

Starting your 1-Day Power Up is so easy, you'll be on the road to overnight weight loss in no time. Here's how you do it.

Important! If you have kidney disease or diabetes, check with your doctor before starting the 1-Day Power Up.

Blender basics

You'll be making three smoothies a day on a weekly basis, and since you may be using frozen fruit or ice in many of them, it's a good idea to choose a durable blender with a strong blade. You can find all kinds of these blenders online – it's worth choosing a good-quality one if you can.

If you're always on the run, look for single-serving blenders that allow you to 'blend and go'. With these space-saving devices, you can just pop off the top, which looks like a glass or sports bottle, and take it with you. Some blenders are so compact that you can fit them into an overnight bag if you're going away or on a business trip. Although convenient, these types of blenders may not have a very sturdy blade, however. This means you may have to introduce ice, frozen foods and denser fruit and veggies little by little to avoid problems, such as the blender grinding to a halt or the blade breaking. With all blenders, you can ensure smoother blending by introducing fruit and veggies in order of density, going from the densest, such as carrots, to the lightest, such as spinach.

Whichever blender you choose, be sure to include the skins of the fruit (except for inedible skins like banana peel) and veggies you use. A lot of the health-promoting and disease-fighting nutrients in produce are found in their skins. Plus, the skin and pulp contain all that good-for-you fibre, which is part of what helps keep you feeling full for hours, keeps your digestive system moving and promotes good health.

Because it is so important that you get this fibre in your smoothies, it is recommended that you avoid using juicers for the 1-Day Power Up. Juicers have gained popularity as a weight-loss tool, but they squeeze out the juice from fruit and vegetables, eliminating the fibre.

Making the 1-Day Power Up smoothies

If you're one of those people who like the ease of following fool-proof instructions, then by all means stick to using the smoothie recipes in Chapter 7. But if you prefer to get a little adventurous, you'll enjoy the option to create your own smoothies using the Mix 'n' Match Smoothie Chart on page 346. That's what Nathalie does.

. . . .

CASE STUDY *Nathalie*

When Nathalie, a 17-year-old student at college, started putting on a lot of weight following puberty, she tried dieting but would get bored with the lack of variety. When she learned that she could create her own smoothies for the 1-Day Power Up, she loved the idea and couldn't wait to start whipping up her own concoctions.

One day, she was trying out a new combo when a couple of her college friends (who weren't dieting) stopped by to see her. She gave them a sample of her smoothie, and they absolutely loved it and asked for more. Now they come over each week on Nathalie's smoothie day as her official 'taste testers'. Together, they've come up with about 30 mixtures of their own. Nathalie, by the way, has lost 2 stone 5 pounds (15kg) and is now at a healthy weight, but still puts her smoothie day into practice.

. . . .

If you want to create your own smoothies, just follow the easy steps here and use the Mix 'n' Match Smoothie Chart on page 346.

1 Choose 1 protein.

2 Choose 1 liquid.

3 Choose up to 2 fruits.

4 Choose up to 3 veggies.

5 Choose up to 2 add-ins (optional).

6 Choose 1 each of as many freebies as you would like (optional).

7 Throw it all into a blender and *voilà*!

THE SIMPLE OPTION

If the thought of taking even a couple of minutes to whip up a delicious smoothie seems too time-consuming, or if you're on the road with no blender in sight, you have yet another option. You can grab my pre-mixed blend that I developed for the Overnight Diet, called Physicians Protein Smoothie. It already includes everything you would throw in the blender, but in a convenient, all-natural powder form that comes in a variety of flavours. Just add water, shake and ta-da! – you've got a flavoured smoothie packed with 20 grams of a proprietary whey-casein protein blend that also includes 5 grams of dietary fibre, plus a host of other ingredients designed to increase satiety, facilitate weight loss and taste great. You can find Physicians Protein Smoothie in good health food stores and on the Overnight Diet website (OvernightDiet.co.uk).

Whether you make your own blend, use the recipes provided, or grab a Physicians Protein Smoothie, these smoothies are delicious. Let's break down what they are made of.

1-Day power up smoothie ingredients

Protein

Adding protein to your smoothies is essential for success on the Overnight Diet and it packs a powerful punch, minimising hunger throughout the day and fuelling lean muscle so that you can boost your metabolism, start burning fat faster and avoid Shrinking Muscle Syndrome. The protein in these smoothies comes from either protein powder or fat-free Greek yogurt.

Protein powders

Protein powders are a powerful way to pump up your protein intake on your smoothie feast day. These are derived from a number of sources and come in a wide variety of flavours. But be aware that some powders contain sweeteners, so be sure to check the sugar content on the nutrition label and to choose one with fewer than 2g of sugar per serving. With a dizzying array of products on the market it can seem a bit confusing, but don't worry, the homework has already been done for you. The best type of protein powder for the Overnight Diet is a whey-casein blend. Other types of protein powders recommended for the Overnight Diet are whey protein isolate and soya protein isolate. These can be found at some supermarkets, in health stores and online.

Whey-casein protein blend For the purposes of this diet, the best protein powder option is a blend of whey and casein. Whey protein is fast digesting and has high levels of leucine, a potent amino acid that stimulates protein synthesis. But this positive effect on protein synthesis is short-lived, and it does not affect protein breakdown. Casein is the most abundant protein in milk. It is processed in such a way that it has a slower rate of digestion, which results in a slow but steady release of amino acids into the bloodstream. One study showed that consuming casein protein resulted in a 34 per cent reduction in protein breakdown. Since whey rapidly increases protein synthesis, and casein blocks protein breakdown, the combination of these two proteins is ideal. It also has little taste, unlike the strong taste of soya protein powders. Research shows that consuming a whey-casein protein mix supports increases in lean body mass and decreases in body fat as part of a resistance-training programme. My proprietary, all natural, whey-casein blend, which I developed for the Overnight Diet, called Physicians Protein Mix, is available in good health food stores and on the Overnight Diet website (OvernightDiet. co.uk). You can use it in any of the smoothie recipes in this book or use it when creating your own smoothies.

Whey protein isolate Whey protein is a high-quality protein derived from cow's milk. Heat processing removes most of the fat and lactose. This type of protein powder contains high levels of branched-chain amino acids, which are the body's natural building blocks for protein. They play an important role in preserving lean muscle and in quelling hunger. Researchers presenting evidence at the Obesity Society Annual Meeting reported that overweight and obese men and women who consumed 60g per day of whey protein for six months had decreased concentrations of the hunger hormone ghrelin.

Soya protein isolate Derived from the soya bean, soya protein is ideal for people who prefer a plant-based protein. Soya protein is virtually carbohydrate-free and fat-free, and like whey protein, it contains all the essential amino acids needed for building protein. Some scientific research has associated soya protein with a reduced risk of heart disease, osteoporosis and some cancers; for example, new research recommends up to two servings a day of soya protein for the prevention of the recurrence of breast cancer. And men, if you think that eating soya foods will give you man-boobs, it won't! That's a myth.

GET THE LOWDOWN ON THE SCIENCE

Making the case for adding omega-3 to your smoothies

There is a growing body of evidence suggesting that increasing your intake of omega-3 fatty acids can reduce body weight and body fat if you're overweight or obese. Not only that, but omega-3 fatty acids can also reduce post-meal hunger, which means they can help keep your stomach from

→

grumbling in between smoothies. Additional research points to a synergistic effect when you increase consumption of omega-3 fatty acids and engage in exercise – increasing the formation of lean muscle and bypassing the storage of excess calories in adipose tissue. That's all great, but who wants to put foul-tasting liquid omega-3 supplements into a smoothie? A better alternative is flaxseed, the richest source of the plant-based omega-3 fatty acid alpha-linolenic acid, which has a mild nutty flavour that tastes great in smoothies. That's why you'll find flaxseeds in several of the smoothie recipes (as well as in the Physicians Protein Smoothie and the Physicians Protein Mix).

When it comes to yogurt, go Greek

Gram for gram, compared to other types of yogurt, Greek yogurt contains almost twice the amount of protein. A typical 175g serving will provide 15–20g of protein, which is about the same amount you would get from 55–85g of chicken breast. That makes it ideal for maintaining lean muscle. Greek yogurt also boasts more probiotics, the biologically active cultures that aid digestion and boost immune support. Plus, even the fat-free versions are thicker and creamier, which makes them more satisfying than other varieties. And because Greek yogurt is strained to remove much of the lactose, it is less likely to be an issue for people who are lactose-intolerant.

This doesn't mean that you can't use other types of yogurt. If your taste buds absolutely refuse to go Greek, find a yogurt you like instead. Just make sure to choose a fat-free or 1 per cent low-fat variety that is low in sugar (12g or less per 175g serving), which means skipping the kind that has the fruit at the bottom. And remember that you may also need to toss in some protein powder to make up for the lower amount of protein in other yogurts.

Look for yogurt with live cultures

If you want to maintain a healthy digestive system, opt for yogurt that contains live cultures. These products are usually natural yogurts and will have the words 'Live' or 'Active Cultures' on the carton. This means the yogurt is a great source of 'good' bacteria, known as probiotics, which help to balance the natural bacteria in your intestines. The most common probiotic found in yogurt is *Lactobacillus acidophilus*. Probiotics may help reduce gas, diarrhoea, cramping and the symptoms of irritable bowel syndrome (IBS). There is also some evidence that they may prevent or minimise vaginal yeast infections as well as the symptoms of colds and flu.

Liquid

When making your smoothies, you can use skimmed milk, your favourite fat-free or low-fat dairy-free alternative, tasty juice, or just water, as well as ice – it's up to you. If you opt for juice, use less than you would if you were using the other liquids. Juice packs more calories and sugar without any protein or any of the heart-healthy fibre you get when eating the whole fruit.

Dairy-free options

If you have problems digesting milk or you would just like to try an alternative to milk, there are a lot of great options, including:

Soya milk Many people are drinking soya milk for its health benefits. Derived from soya beans, it is high in protein and contains more fibre than regular milk. It also contains soya isoflavones, which have been linked to reducing the risk of heart disease, cancer and osteoporosis. It has been found to reduce menopause symptoms in some women. Cholesterol-free and low in saturated fat, soya milk also provides vitamin D and calcium.

Almond milk is becoming more and more popular. The fact that it is low in calories, low in cholesterol, low in salt and low in sugar explains part of its appeal. Plus, it has healthy doses of calcium, and vitamins D, E and A, so it's easy to see why people are giving it a try. When choosing almond milk, opt for an unsweetened variety.

Coconut milk Coconuts and coconut milk were once considered diet disasters, because they contain natural saturated fats. But emerging research has found that the type of saturated fat in coconuts is rapidly used as energy rather than being stored as fat. Even so, choose light coconut milk rather than the full-fat version to reduce the calorie content. It contains vitamins and minerals that support the immune system. Note that coconut milk and coconut water are not one and the same. Coconut milk is derived from squeezing the flesh of the coconut. The clear liquid that drains from the fruit is coconut water.

GET THE LOWDOWN ON THE SCIENCE

Why the fat in coconut milk won't make you fat

Not all saturated fat is created equal. Coconuts and coconut milk are rich in medium-chain fatty acids (MCFAs), a type of saturated fat that is quickly metabolised by the liver. This means the body rapidly burns it as fuel rather than sending it to your fat cells for storage. Compare that to long-chain fatty acids (LCFAs), which are the saturated fats typically found in meats and dairy products. Research on animals has shown that LCFAs are more likely to wind up as fat on the body. In a few small human studies, people eating a diet rich in MCFAs had higher metabolisms than those consuming LCFAs.

Fruit

You can use fresh fruit, canned fruit or frozen fruit (un-sweetened). If you use canned fruit, make sure the fruit is canned in its own juice rather than syrup, and always drain the juice first. Filled with disease-fighting antioxidants, fruit is also a good source of fibre that helps you feel full longer, so you won't get the munchies 20 minutes after you finish your smoothie. On the Overnight Diet, *all* fruits are acceptable.

Non-starchy veggies

Use fresh vegetables whenever possible, but you can also use frozen or canned veggies at a pinch. One of the coolest things about sneaking veggies into smoothies is that they pack a powerful nutrition punch while adding healthy fibre. But the best thing is that you can't even taste them – great if you've never been a big fan of spinach or kale!

. . . .

CASE STUDY *Emily*

Veggies didn't bother Emily, a university student who at 23 years of age had already successfully lost 1 stone 4 pounds (8.2kg), but she had hit a plateau and just couldn't get rid of those last 10 pounds (4.5kg). When she heard about the 1-Day Power Up and how it helps break through plateaus, she was eager to try it. Fortunately, she arrived at the Nutrition and Weight Management Center at Boston Medical Center on a day when several smoothies were being subjected to a taste test. Emily was told she could pick one to try. 'I love chocolate,' she said, and zeroed in on the Spa Crazy Chocolate smoothie (page 188). After a few sips, Emily gave it a big thumbs up. 'What's in it?' she asked. When she saw the list of ingredients, which included spinach, Emily almost fell out of her chair. 'You're joking! There's no way this can have spinach in it. I *hate* spinach,' she said.

. . . .

As you'll discover, adding veggies is a sneaky way to get more fibre without significantly altering the taste of the smoothie. As for Emily, she now throws in handfuls of spinach knowing she'll get lots of great nutrients without having to taste it. And she adds, 'I wish my mum would have been smart enough to give me my veggies this way.'

Add-ins (optional)

Here's where you can really have some fun with your smoothies. Think chocolate syrup, peanut butter, molasses and more! Some of the Add-Ins (see page 347) may seem a little out of the ordinary to you, but they are delicious, and all of them boast health benefits. But remember that add-ins are optional; it's completely up to you whether to include them or not.

Freebies (optional)

On page 347 you will find a list of flavourings, spices, sugar substitutes and other goodies that can really make your smoothie your own. If you love cinnamon or nutmeg, sprinkle away! Love iced coffee? Try adding brewed coffee to create a mocha latte smoothie. It's up to you.

Spice up your smoothies with added flavour

Turning your smoothies into fun, fanciful creations is easy. Flavourings and extracts as well as spices from your kitchen cupboards can transform an ordinary smoothie into something extraordinary. With all of these, a little goes a long way; you only need to use a small amount to get a big taste: ¼–½ tsp of spices and ¼–1 tsp of flavourings and extracts. The latter may contain calories and sweeteners, but because you'll be using such small doses, the amounts are negligible. In terms of flavourings and extracts, you can use traditional ones like vanilla extract, chocolate, orange, lemon or lime. But if you really want to get creative, there are many unique, tasty flavours you can find. The same goes for spices. The Smoothie Flavourings and Extracts list on page 348 and the Smoothie Spices list also on page 348 will give you plenty of ideas. If you can't find the ones you want in your local supermarket, you can find a wide selection online.

Sweet success

If you like a little sweetness in your coffee or tea, two no-calorie sweeteners that are recommended on the Overnight Diet are Truvia, which is made with stevia, and Splenda, which is also known as sucralose. You can find Truvia and Splenda in just about any supermarket. Stevia is just catching on as a sugar substitute. If you can't find it in your local supermarket, you can order it online.

Revel in some rest and relaxation

When you get started on the Overnight Diet, you'll first choose one day of the week to be your weekly 1-Day Power Up day. Pick the day that will work best for you consistently – it doesn't matter which day that is. Many people choose Sunday because they don't have to work and are at home where they have all their smoothie ingredients at hand.

Another reason people love the 1-Day Power Up so much is because in addition to jump-starting the metabolic processes that induce overnight weight loss, it can also act as a wind-down rest and relaxation day. You have permission to take a break from physical activity – if you want to – and luxuriate with a day of rest and relaxation. Think of how a plug-in hybrid electric car is charged while in the 'off' mode, restoring the energy it spent on its last trip and juicing up for its next. That's what this transitional and transformational day can do for you: rejuvenate and recharge.

On the very first day you start the Overnight Diet, the 1-Day Power Up will be doing just that – powering up your body for the coming week. On subsequent 1-Day Power Up days, you will not only be charging up for the coming week but also taking a breather from the previous week's 6-Day Fuel Up. Think of the rest and relaxation aspect of this day as a spa day when you get to pamper yourself and enjoy some well-deserved 'me time'. Do your best to take it easy. Here are some of the ways my weight-loss patients choose to unwind:

'I turn on some calming music while I'm going about my day.'

'I sit on the sofa and watch football.'

'I like to do some gentle stretching.'

'I take a nap in the afternoon. What a luxury!'

'I spend time with friends.'

Taking a respite from your hectic life can do wonders for your mood and help you de-stress, which is yet another way the 1-Day Power Up works to encourage weight loss. Mountains of scientific evidence have identified a strong link between stress and weight gain and, in particular, with an increase in belly fat. In fact, women who have slender arms, legs and hips but fat around the abdomen have been found to have high levels of the stress hormone cortisol. Feeling frazzled day in and day out raises levels of the stress hormone cortisol, which wreaks havoc with your weight. It can slow your metabolism, cause your body to store fat around the abdominal organs, affect your blood sugar levels, reduce levels of the body's muscle-building hormones and increase cravings. To put it simply, stress leads to weight gain, emotional eating and Shrinking Muscle Syndrome. Taking advantage of the weekly 1-Day Power Up to relax and rejuvenate can help reverse this process.

....

CASE STUDY *Karen*

Just ask Karen, a 40-year-old working mother of three, who had about 2 stone 2 pounds (13.6kg) to lose. Karen was so busy with her job, housework and shuttling her kids to and from school and activities that she felt stressed all the time. She wanted to lose weight but she didn't have a lot of time to devote to a diet with lots of complicated recipes or a lengthy initiation phase. She wanted a quick and easy method to lose weight, and she wanted fast results – like tomorrow! She loved the idea of overnight weight loss that lasts, and was eager to get started.

Fast forward to one of her follow-up appointments, and Karen was thrilled that she was quickly zeroing in on her goal. That's not unusual on this diet, but then Karen explained how the 1-Day Power Up had literally changed her life.

Karen said that turning it into a weekly rest and relaxation day had helped her learn how to relax and de-stress. Just taking some time out for herself on that one day per week allowed her to recharge her batteries so she didn't feel so run-down and crazed all the time. 'I think I had forgotten how to relax and pamper myself,' she said. 'And I really needed to rediscover that.'

....

What is more, the 1-Day Power Up also made Karen completely re-evaluate her relationship with food. She quickly realised that she had been using food as a way to self-soothe: to calm her when she felt stressed; to boost her mood when she felt sad, mad or anxious; and to give her something to do when she was bored. It was also a form of entertainment for her. Every family outing revolved around food – going out to dinner, stopping for a celebratory treat after one of the kid's football matches, filling up on popcorn and fizzy drinks at the cinema. Every get-together with her girlfriends, like her monthly book group meeting, involved lots of fattening foods or cocktails, and sometimes both. Every work event she attended turned into a food foray, too.

'It was like I couldn't survive more than an hour without eating something,' Karen said. 'I was convinced that I was going to be starving on the 1-Day Power Up. But when I actually tried it, I wasn't hungry at all in between my smoothies. I couldn't believe it. Throughout the rest of the week, I started paying attention to the times when I would feel hungry, and it finally dawned on me that most of the time when I would eat, it rarely had anything to do with actually being hungry. That was an eye-opener for me.'

GET THE LOWDOWN ON THE SCIENCE

De-stress to weigh less

Reducing stress is one of the key ingredients for weight loss, according to a study appearing in a 2011 issue of the *International Journal of Obesity*. A team of scientists from Kaiser Permanente Center for Health Research, in the US, enlisted almost 500 participants and asked them to lose at least 10 pounds (4.5kg) in six months. The volunteers were also asked to report on their stress levels in addition to their sleep habits, moods and more. The results showed that participants with the lowest stress levels who got at least six but not more than eight hours of sleep were the most likely to lose at least 10 pounds (4.5kg). In fact they were twice as likely to have lost 10 pounds (4.5kg) or more than the people who reported the highest stress levels and got less than six hours of shut-eye on a regular basis.

Tales of the Measuring Tape

'I don't cook, so I love the smoothie day. It's so easy, even I can do it.' Joseph, 56, lost 3 stone 5 pounds (21.3kg)

A lot of people experience this kind of breakthrough just by practising the 1-Day Power Up. With this diet, though, you don't have to do any deep soul-searching about the emotional reasons why you overeat; you don't have to keep a food diary; and you don't have to start writing down your every thought and emotion. However, gaining an awareness of your appetite can help you get in tune with your body's hunger and satiety signals. Engaging in some simple mindful-eating habits is one way to do so. Here are a few tips:

- Before you eat, ask yourself, 'Am I really hungry?'

- Sit down to eat your meals or drink your smoothie, as opposed to standing.

- Don't watch TV, read the newspaper, or check your email while dining.

- Savour your food – or smoothie – rather than wolfing it down.

- Eat as if others were watching you; in public, you probably wouldn't stuff your face, for example.

- Eat – or drink – until you are satisfied. On a scale of 1–10, with 1 being ravenous and 10 being post-Christmas-dinner full, aim for a 7 (not still hungry, but not stuffed either).

The 1-Day Power Up can go a long way towards changing the way you eat – for the better! It helped Karen change some of the food habits that were contributing to that extra 2 stone 2 pounds (13.6kg) she had been carrying around. Initially Karen thought she couldn't go to her book group meeting because it was her smoothie day. That if she wasn't going to partake in the big plate of biscuits they always ate, somehow she wasn't participating in the group. But then she realised she should just take her smoothie with her to book group.

So Karen arrived one night to her book group with one of her own smoothie creations – a tropical concoction with a banana-flavoured protein powder, light coconut milk and mango. Her friends were so impressed with her new slimmed-down appearance that they wanted to know what she was drinking and wanted the recipe too. So the next time she hosted the book group, Karen decided to make smoothies instead of putting out the usual spread of biscuits. Her friends loved it! Now, their book group night has become a smoothie night. And some of the other women in the group have started following the Overnight Diet and losing weight with Karen.

The simple yet powerful realisation that she didn't have to be a slave to her old eating habits at her book group led to other lifestyle changes for Karen, which, when combined with her 1-Day Power Up and 6-Day Fuel Up, sparked even speedier weight loss. And it has helped her keep that weight off. Karen reached her goal weight three years ago, and hasn't gained a pound since.

Tales of the Measuring Tape

'Having a rest and relaxation day is the best. Carving out a day of "me" time each Sunday allows my body, and my mind, to get the rest it needs. Then when Monday comes along, I feel energised and ready to go for the week.'
Nina, 31, lost 1½ stone (9.5kg) and has kept it off for 19 months

Power Up and prep

The 1-Day Power Up also serves as an ideal preparation day to get ready for the coming 6-Day Fuel Up. It's a great time to review the meal plan for the coming week, to ensure that your fridge is stocked with the good-for-you foods you will be eating on the 6-Day Fuel Up, to prepare snacks so that you can just grab them and go, and to prepare any recipes that might taste better if made a day or two before consuming them. That way, when you come home from work in the evenings, everything's all ready to go. You don't have to worry about what you're going to make, and you don't have to run to the shop for ingredients you don't have.

....

6-Day Fuel Up

If you have already completed your 1-Day Power Up, congratulations! You are up to 2 pounds (900g) lighter, and you have revved up your body's fat-burning process. The next six days are the key to keeping up the momentum so that you can continue to burn fat and lose up to 9 pounds (4kg) in the first week.

As I have already pointed out, the foundation of the 6-Day Fuel Up lies in a diet plan first used in a medical setting. But for a diet to be effective long term, it can't just produce results in the lab or in a medically supervised environment. It has to work in the crazy reality we call life, where on some days you have mere minutes to get the entire family fed and out the door in the morning and then you have just 15 minutes to whip up dinner in the evening. Rest assured, the 6-Day Fuel Up has been developed with real people in mind and has been engineered to produce maximum results safely *and* be easy enough to follow that it works in the real world, without any necessary doctor supervision.

You've already learned how it works together with the 1-Day Power Up to maintain fat burning at a high level, how it contributes to the production of lean muscle and how it promotes optimal health. But now you're about to discover why it will be so easy for you to follow:

You won't go hungry The foods you will be eating during these six days have been shown to provide the greatest levels of satiety. This means that they will keep you feeling full the longest. Plus, if you do get the munchies, you can choose from lots of grab-and-go snacks – guilt-free!

You won't feel deprived Many diets bombard you with endless lists of foods to avoid, leaving you with extremely limited choices. When there's next to nothing that you are allowed to eat, it increases the likelihood that you will give up long before you get the results you want. On the Overnight Diet, you won't have that problem. The focus of the 6-Day Fuel Up is on feeding the muscles with adequate protein and fuelling the body with great-tasting, good-for-you foods that will result in rapid fat loss, not deprivation. There is an abundance of delicious foods, and no food group is off limits; you won't even feel like you're dieting. Instead of telling you what to take away, the Overnight Diet lets you add to your plate with unlimited fruit and non-starchy veg.

....

CASE STUDY *Ed*

At 51, Ed loved Indian food, spicy chillies and huge burgers, all of which contributed to the extra 2 stone (12.7kg) of fat he had been carrying around for about 20 years. To trim down, Ed would periodically try some sort of crash diet. He would typically lose about 10 pounds (4.5kg) pretty quickly, but he always felt like he was starving to death, and he was so deprived of all the foods he loved that he could never stick with those drastic plans. After a couple of weeks, he would usually chuck the whole plan out the window and go on a week-long binge, gaining back all 10 pounds (4.5kg) – and a couple more.

When he tried the Overnight Diet, Ed was amazed that he could eat so much food and so many of the foods he loved – with a healthy twist – and still lose weight. He didn't feel deprived, so he found it easy to stay on the plan. He eventually lost those 2 stone (12.7kg) and has kept the weight off for more than two years. See the box to find out what Ed would eat on a typical day on the 6-Day Fuel Up.

ED'S 6-DAY FUEL UP MEALS

Breakfast Egg and Spinach Omelette, an orange and coffee

Snack Baked Cinnamon Apples

Lunch Beefy Mushroom Burger and an apple

Snack Veggies with Avocado-Corn Salsa

Dinner Spicy Chicken & Cannellini Bean Chilli, Baked Cheesy Tomatoes and a glass of wine

Dessert Grandma's Low-fat Chocolate Pudding

Snack Blueberries

You won't get bored With more than 100 lip-smacking foods you can eat right from the start, you won't be forced to eat the same boring fare day in and day out. Variety will keep you engaged and excited while you slim down.

GET THE LOWDOWN ON THE SCIENCE

Variety is the spice of a healthy life

Diets that severely restrict the types of foods you can eat, or that eliminate entire categories of food, may be sabotaging your health, according to University of Arkansas researcher Peter Ungar, author of *Human Diet: Its Origin and Evolution*. Ungar points to evidence suggesting that humans evolved to consume a wider array of foods than any other species. And when it comes to our health, the wider the better. So, instead of narrowing your food choices to a few select approved foods, it is better for your health to enjoy a wide variety of foods like you will on the Overnight Diet. It's guaranteed that you'll like it better too.

You'll love the flexibility If you're running late, you will find foods and meals that you can simply grab on your way out the door. Or if you enjoy getting creative in the kitchen, you can experiment to your heart's content. You also don't have to worry about fitting meals into a rigid schedule. You don't have to eat breakfast at 7.38am, a snack exactly two hours and 12 minutes later, lunch at 12.17pm, another snack exactly three hours and seven minutes later, and then dinner at 6.06pm. Life can get crazy, and a diet has to fit into your schedule in order to work long term, so there is flexibility built into this plan.

You don't have to be an algebra whiz Phew! You can forget about counting calories, adding up points, weighing every serving of food, calculating ratios of macronutrients to put on your plate, or working out percentages of your daily intake. There is only one number you need to know: your DPR, and the charts on pages 85–6 will do the calculating for you.

GET THE LOWDOWN ON THE SCIENCE

Easy does it, complicated doesn't

It may seem obvious, but diets that are more complicated, that involve a lot of rules and requirements and that take up a lot of time are harder to stick with. That means the more complicated a diet is the more likely you are to give up on it without getting the weight-loss benefits you want. This insight comes from a 2010 study in *Appetite*, in which cognitive scientists from Indiana University and the Max Planck Institute for Human Development in Berlin compared how women fared on two very different diet plans. One diet involved very simple meal plans while the other required dieters to calculate every morsel of food they ate. They found that the more complicated people thought their diet plan was, the faster they gave up on it.

There's no guesswork At the Nutrition and Weight Management Center at Boston Medical Center, there is a food storecupboard stocked with all the appropriate foods, so patients can see first-hand what a healthy storecupboard looks like. On page 349, you'll find the Overnight Diet Shopping List to help you create your own Overnight Diet storecupboard. It's easier than you think.

Tales of the Measuring Tape

'I can't tell you how happy I am that I don't have to count calories!' Lynette, 31, lost 1 stone 5 pounds (8.6kg)

You'll love the simplicity On the 6-Day Fuel Up, there are only four simple prescriptions to follow. They aren't time-consuming, they don't require any expensive equipment, and they don't involve complicated food combining. Just four clear, easy-to-follow, fat-blasting, weight-busting prescriptions. And if you follow these, you will see results – fast. Let's look more closely at each of them.

The four ways to faster fat loss

All you have to do is adhere to the following four simple prescriptions and you will be on your way to a whole new you, including a slimmer, trimmer and stronger body.

Prescription no. 1: meet your DPR every day

Meeting your Daily Protein Requirement (DPR) is an indispensable component of the 6-Day Fuel Up. Getting adequate protein each day not only preserves lean muscle to boost metabolism and prevent Shrinking Muscle Syndrome but it also prevents hunger pangs. As you have seen, protein rates high in terms of satiety, meaning it keeps you feeling full for hours. When you are eating the proper amount of protein, your stomach won't be grumbling. Here's how to find your DPR:

Daily Protein Requirement (DPR):
Ideal weight (in kilograms) × 1.5g = DPR

So the first step to calculating your DPR is to find your ideal weight in the charts on pages 85–6. At the Nutrition and Weight Management Center at Boston Medical Center, a complex formula is used to determine each individual's ideal weight, but this has been simplified for you here. For women, ideal weight is calculated as 7 stone (44.5kg) for the first 5 feet (1.5m) in height and an additional 5 pounds (2.25kg) for every 1 inch (2.5cm) over 5 feet (1.5m); for men, it is 7½ stone (47.6kg) for the first 5 feet (1.5m) in height and an additional 6 pounds (2.7kg) for every 1 inch (2.5cm) over 5 feet (1.5m). After you find your ideal weight on the chart, simply read across: the figure given in the next column is the amount of protein you need to eat per day, your DPR; the final column provides your DPR in terms of the amount of *protein-rich food* – that's lean meat, fish, poultry, eggs, soya products, meat substitutes and protein powder – you need to eat per day in order to achieve that intake. Protein-rich foods are not solely made up of protein – there is about 7g of protein in every 28g (1 ounce) of meat, poultry or fish. This means, for example, that you would need to eat 140g of fish in order to take in 35g of protein. (It's a little more complicated for the vegetarian sources of protein that count towards your DPR, but the chart on page 88 outlines how much each of these sources contribute towards your daily total.) The purpose of the final column is to save you doing the maths. Note: the recipes that contribute to your DPR give the 'Protein per serving towards DPR' – this is the contribution to your daily total of protein-rich food.

Remember your DPR figures or write them down – it's vital that you meet this minimum intake. There is one caveat, however: even if your ideal weight is below 8 stone 8 pounds (54.4kg), your minimum DPR will still be 82g and therefore 350g of lean protein foods per day. Eating less protein than that can be dangerous, no matter how petite you are.

Here's an example of how this equation works. Let's say you are a 5ft 9in (1.75m) male. According to the chart on page 86, your ideal weight is 11 stone 6 pounds (72.5kg). Now look across the chart to find your DPR (109g). This means consuming 450g of meat, fish, poultry, eggs or high-protein vegetarian food per day. Remember, this is just an example. You must determine your individual DPR to make the Overnight Diet work for you.

Find Your DPR (for women)

Find your height on the left then read across to find your ideal weight and DPR/daily total of meat, fish, poultry, eggs or high-protein vegetarian food.

Height	Ideal weight	DPR	DPR (minimum quantity of protein-rich food needed per day)
5ft 4in (1.62m)	up to 8 stone 8lb (54.4kg)	82g	350g
5ft 5in (1.65m)	8 stone 13lb (56.7kg)	85g	350g
5ft 6in (1.67m)	9 stone 4lb (58.9kg)	89g	375g
5ft 7in (1.70m)	9 stone 9lb (61.2kg)	92g	375g
5ft 8in (1.72m)	10 stone (63.5kg)	95g	400g
5ft 9in (1.75m)	10 stone 5lb (65.7kg)	99g	400g
5ft 10in (1.77m)	10 stone 10lb (68kg)	102g	425g
5ft 11in (1.80m)	11 stone 1lb (70.3kg)	105g	425g
6ft (1.83m)	11 stone 6lb (72.5kg)	109g	450g
6ft 1in (1.85m)	11 stone 11lb (74.8kg)	112g	450g
6ft 2in (1.88m)	12 stone 2lb (77.1kg)	116g	475g

Find Your DPR (for men)

Find your height on the left then read across to find your ideal weight and DPR/daily total of meat, fish, poultry, eggs or high-protein vegetarian food.

Height	Ideal weight	DPR	DPR (minimum quantity of protein-rich food needed per day)
up to 5ft 6in (1.67m)	up to 10 stone 2lb (54.4kg)	97g	400g
5ft 7in (1.70m)	10 stone 8lb (67.1kg)	101g	400g
5ft 8in (1.72m)	11 stone (69.3kg)	105g	425g
5ft 9in (1.75m)	11 stone 6lb (72.5kg)	109g	450g
5ft 10in (1.77m)	11 stone 12lb (75.2kg)	113g	450g
5ft 11in (1.80m)	12 stone 4lb (78kg)	117g	480g
6ft (1.83m)	12 stone 10lb (80.7kg)	121g	480g
6ft 1in (1.85m)	13 stone 2lb (83.4kg)	125g	500g
6ft 2in (1.88m)	13 stone 8lb (86.1kg)	129g	500g
6ft 3in (1.90m)	14 stone 1lb (88.9kg)	133g	540g
6ft 4in (1.93m)	14 stone 6lb (91.6kg)	137g	570g
6ft 6in (1.98m)	14 stone 12lb (94.3kg)	141g	570g

Tales of the Measuring Tape

'I thought I was eating enough protein, but I suppose I wasn't. Since I upped my protein intake, I've definitely noticed a difference in my body composition – less fat and more toned. I love it!' Leslie, lost 12 pounds (5.4kg) and 2½ inches (6cm) off her waist

Getting adequate protein for your individual needs is a cornerstone of this programme. It's what fuels your muscles and boosts metabolism. Getting the right type of protein is also important. In general, when it comes to protein, the leaner the better. On the 6-Day Fuel Up, you must meet your minimum DPR from your choice of the following lean protein sources: lean beef, lean pork, poultry and fish; eggs; soya products, meat alternatives and protein powder.

Other protein sources do not count towards your DPR. This means that even though this eating plan recommends 2 servings daily of fat-free or low-fat dairy and up to 1 serving daily of legumes and pulses such as lentils, chickpeas and black-eyed beans, the protein in these foods does *not* count towards your DPR. Why not? In addition to containing protein, these foods contain carbohydrates and natural sugars, which react differently in the body and do not provide the same level of muscle-preserving, fat-burning benefits compared to the more pure protein sources listed overleaf. This is why these foods are limited to the number of servings indicated. Overleaf is a list of lean protein options that are recommended for the 6-Day Fuel Up.

Figuring out how much protein to eat to meet your daily total of protein foods is easy if you're choosing meat or fish because, for example, 30g of these protein sources equals 30g towards your total daily intake. But what about eggs, tofu and other sources? Use the chart overleaf as a reference tool.

Protein sources that count towards your DPR for the 6-Day Fuel Up

Lean beef	thick flank or top rump, topside and silverside, fillet steak
Lean pork	pork chops, pork loin
Fish	cod, haddock, halibut, other white fish; mackerel, salmon, tuna steak and other oily fish; canned tuna/salmon/sardines in water
Poultry	skinless light meat chicken and turkey
Eggs	hard-boiled, soft-boiled, poached, pan-fried with non-stick cooking spray
Soya products and meat alternatives	tofu, tempeh, seitan, TVP
Protein powder	Physicians Protein Mix, whey, soya

Contribution of protein sources towards total DPR

Protein source	Protein towards DPR
30g lean beef	30g
30g lean pork	30g
30g fish	30g
30g poultry	30g
1 large egg	30g
2 large egg whites	30g
85g tofu	30g
45g tempeh	30g
30g seitan	30g
2 tbsp TVP	30g
⅓ scoop protein powder approx.	30g (check label)

Can I do The Overnight Diet if I'm a vegetarian?

Yes! It is easier than you might think to meet your DPR with soya products, meat alternatives and eggs. If you're a vegetarian or a vegan, you can replace poultry, pork or beef in the recipes in the meal plan with tofu, seitan or tempeh, though you must ensure you use the correct amount to meet your DPR (see the chart opposite). Another meat substitute is textured vegetable protein (TVP), which is made from dried soya protein. All you have to do is place equal parts TVP and boiling water into a measuring cup, wait 5 minutes, and it's ready to go. For meals that call for bacon or sausage, you can use veggie versions of these products, which can be found in most supermarkets. In recipes that call for chicken or beef stock, feel free to use vegetable stock instead. If you're concerned about consuming soya products, rest assured that decades of research have shown that soya products are associated with numerous health benefits.

JUST SAY NO: HIGHER-FAT PROTEIN SOURCES

You should avoid the following higher-fat protein sources because dietary fats can be a contributing factor in insulin resistance and inflammation, both of which promote weight gain and obesity.

- **Higher-fat meats** Regular minced beef, prime cuts or heavily marbled meats, spare ribs, goose, duck, wild game, organ meats.

- **Processed meats** Bacon, sausage, corned beef, hot dogs, luncheon meats, hams and other cold cuts with more than 3g fat per 25g.

- **Dairy** Whole milk, full-fat yogurt, full-fat cheeses, cream.

Prescription no. 2: Stick to lean carbs

You can enjoy a selection of all-you-can-eat fruit and non-starchy vegetables, up to 100g of starchy veggies, and 2–3 servings of whole grains absolutely guilt-free.

You should enjoy an abundant variety of lean carbs: high-fibre, heart-healthy, disease-fighting foods. Lean carbs are the good-for-you carbs that will help you lose the muffin top or love handles and keep them off. Remember, research shows that people who eat the most lean carbs are the least likely to be over-weight or obese – but they must be the right carbs. It's time to stop feeling guilty for eating fruit or having a slice of wholemeal bread and start enjoying them again. Your body will thank you for it.

Savour all of the fruit and non-starchy vegetables you want from your 'all-you-can-eat' selection. When was the last time you got the green light to enjoy 'all you can eat' of anything? Avoiding hunger pangs is essential when trying to lose weight; endless fruit and veggies ensures that you will never go hungry. Think fruit and veggies are boring? The Spice Up Your Veggies chart and the Spice Up Your Fruit chart in Appendix B offer tips on how to turn ordinary produce into something extraordinary.

Does this mean you can't have any starchy veggies on the 6-Day Fuel Up? No, it doesn't. Although your three snacks a day will be made up solely of fruit and non-starchy veggies, your meals can include these as well as up to 100g of starchy veggies a day, including sweetcorn, potatoes, sweet potatoes and squash.

The fibre factor

Staving off hunger is only one of the reasons why this diet places such a strong emphasis on lean carbs, fruit and vegetables. That high satiety factor is achieved in large part thanks to all the healthy fibre they contain. And fibre contributes to better health in a number of ways, which include:

- Reducing hunger
- Reducing cholesterol
- Reducing the risk of heart disease and stroke
- Reducing the risk of cancer
- Reducing the risk of type-2 diabetes
- Helping maintain optimal kidney function
- Improving bowel function

But remember, much of the fibre – as well as the vitamins and minerals – is found in the skin of fruit and vegetables, so eat them without peeling when possible. Of course, you have to peel bananas and oranges, but it's best to eat apples, pears, cucumbers and other fruits and vegetables with the skin on for a quick fibre boost.

Quick shopping tip for fruit and vegetables Fresh produce makes great snacks, but it can spoil if you don't eat it soon enough. It's a good idea to keep canned and frozen fruit and vegetables so that you will always have them to hand. When buying canned, choose fruit in water or in its own juice rather than in syrup, and look for canned vegetables that aren't loaded with salt. With frozen foods, opt for fruit without added sugar and vegetables without butter or cream sauces.

This plan is formulated to help you lose weight in a way that promotes good health rather than endangering it. There is a veritable bounty of health benefits that come from eating fruit and vegetables. Why are these foods such powerful disease fighters? Think of your body for a moment as if it is a big factory. Inside your factory, your cells – which are like the employees on your production line – are hard at work every moment of every day converting oxygen to energy. But each time they do so, they create a by-product: molecules called free radicals. Think of free radicals as Ninja assassins that race through your body's factory damaging and destroying the equipment – the proteins, tissues and genes. The work of these Ninja assassins is associated with many diseases, including cancer and heart disease. To counter-attack the Ninja assassins, your body relies on an army of soldiers called antioxidants. Like superheroes, antioxidants neutralise the Ninjas so that your body's equipment can keep operating at full steam.

Where does your body get antioxidants? From fruit and veg-etables! Unfortunately, many people eat only 59 per cent of the daily recommended amount of vegetables and 42 per cent of fruit. The Overnight Diet aims to counteract this problem by encouraging you to eat abundant amounts of them, which help to fight disease and keep your body in peak condition. Plus, with dozens of fruits and vegetables from which to choose, you will never get bored. The name of the game on this diet is variety, not deprivation. Have a look at the Overnight Diet Shopping List (Appendix B) to see the many fruits and vegetables you can enjoy while burning fat and losing weight, as well as the list of fruits and veggies that are high in antioxidants.

Eat 2–3 servings of whole grains per day

Another important way to get lean carbs is through whole grains. On this diet, you have permission to eat delicious foods like wholemeal bread, oats, wholewheat pasta and brown rice. Whole grains are those containing 100 per cent of the entire grain kernel, including the bran, germ and endosperm. Whole grains also contain fibre, vitamins, minerals and antioxidants. Refined grains, on the other hand, go through a process to remove the bran and germ. The refining process also removes fibre and nutrients.

Carbohydrates have been vilified in the past, but whole grains are an essential part of a healthy diet. That's why dozens of respected health organisations in the US, UK and Australia advocate eating whole grains. Decades of scientific evidence have shown that doing so has been associated with a number of health benefits, which include:

- Reducing the risk of heart disease by 25–28 per cent
- Reducing the risk of diabetes by 21–30 per cent
- Reducing the risk of stroke by 30–36 per cent
- Reducing the risk of metabolic syndrome
- Reducing insulin levels and insulin resistance
- Reducing blood glucose levels
- Reducing total cholesterol
- Reducing LDL cholesterol
- Raising HDL cholesterol
- Reducing triglycerides
- Reducing C-reactive protein, an inflammation marker
- Reducing the risk of inflammatory disease
- Promoting healthier arteries
- Lowering the risk of colorectal cancer
- Reducing blood pressure levels
- Reducing the risk of asthma
- Promoting healthier gums and teeth

Add to this list of remarkable health benefits the fact that a diet rich in whole grains contributes to weight loss. Between 2004 and 2009 alone, there were at least ten studies showing that whole grains promote weight loss, reduce BMI and, in particular, reduce waist circumference. Combine all these benefits, and it's easy to see that whole grains make a whole lot of sense for healthy weight loss.

But how does eating whole-grain breads, cereals, rice and pasta help you get slim and stay slim? For one thing, whole grains are jam-packed with fibre to promote satiety and tune down the hunger hormone ghrelin. A study in the *European Journal of Endocrinology* showed that eating a diet high in fibre helps balance ghrelin levels in people carrying extra pounds. That spells hunger relief.

GET THE LOWDOWN ON THE SCIENCE

Eat whole grains to whittle your waist

Here are just a few of the many highlights from research showing the relationship between whole grains and weight loss.

A team of researchers from Penn State put two groups of people on the same diet, which included five daily servings of fruit and vegetables, three servings of low-fat dairy products and two servings of lean protein. The only difference in the diet was that one group ate only whole grains while the other group ate refined grains. After 12 weeks, both groups lost an average of 8–11 pounds (3.6–5kg), but the group eating whole grains lost significantly more abdominal fat. Wouldn't you like a trimmer waist so that you can wear a smaller size?

In the *Journal of the American College of Nutrition*, researchers investigated the relationship between BMI and whole-grain consumption in women. They found that women who consumed at least one serving of whole grains per day had a significantly lower BMI and waist measurement than women who consumed no whole grains.

In a study of 159 college students appearing in the *Journal of Nutrition and Education Behavior*, researchers found

→

that whole grain intake was highest among students with a healthy weight and lower among those who were overweight or obese.

When researchers from the Netherlands analysed whole-grain consumption among 4,237 middle-aged adults, they reported in the *European Journal of Nutrition* that for each additional gram of whole-grain consumption in both men and women, the risk of being obese was lower.

6-Day Fuel Up whole-grain serving sizes

If you think a serving of whole-grain cereal is whatever fits into the giant bowl you took out of the cupboard, think again. In our society, we often overestimate serving sizes, and this is one of the problems leading to overeating and weight gain. So, what constitutes a serving size? Look at the following list for accurate serving sizes:

- Half a 100 per cent wholemeal bagel
- 1 thin slice 100 per cent wholemeal bread (1 serving = 30g)
- 140g oats, cooked (or 30g raw)
- 1 serving ready-to-eat, high-fibre cereal (1 serving as per nutrition label)
- 80g brown rice, cooked (or 30g raw)
- 100g wholemeal pasta, cooked (or 30g raw)
- 80g couscous, cooked (or 30g raw)
- 95g quinoa, cooked (or 30g raw)
- 2 whole-grain crackers

Prescription no. 3: focus on healthy fats; limit added fats to 4 servings per day

Just as all carbohydrates are not created equal, neither are all fats. In the West, most of us consume too many fatty foods: we eat 280 per cent of the recommended amount of solid fats and sugars and 110 per cent of saturated fats. This is bad news for our waistlines and for our health. For decades, saturated fats have been associated with increased risk of cardiovascular disease. A seminal study published in the *New England Journal of Medicine* reported that each increase of 5 per cent of calories from saturated fat as compared with equivalent intake from carbohydrates was associated with a 17 per cent increase in risk of heart disease. Pretty scary stuff, but the question doctors everywhere were asking was, 'What do we use to replace the saturated fat?'

Most of the low-fat diets designed in response to these findings allowed free rein to eat carbohydrates in place of those nasty saturated fats, but did not differentiate between whole-grain and refined carbs. As you now know, eating too many refined carbohydrates has also been found to increase the risk of heart disease and diabetes. In fact, they may be even more detrimental to your health than saturated fats. That makes things a little confusing, doesn't it?

Doctors, scientists and researchers went back to the drawing board and headed back to their labs to do more research. And there have been some important revelations. The message about ditching refined carbohydrates in favour of lean carbs like the Overnight Diet recommends is coming through crystal clear. But what about those fats? Do all types of fat contribute to disease? Or are saturated fats the only villains? Do all fats go immediately to your thighs and belly? Do you have to eliminate all fats if you want to burn fat?

The exciting news is that while overeating saturated fats promotes disease and weight gain, eating certain types of fats in the right amounts might actually help you burn fat and promote better health. What are these potential fat-burning, disease-fighting fats?

Say hello to PUFAs and MUFAs

PUFAs are polyunsaturated fatty acids. Unlike saturated fats, which are solid at room temperature, PUFAs are typically in liquid form whether at room temperature or chilled. PUFAs contain essential fatty acids (EFAs) called omega-3 fatty acids and omega-6 fatty acids. Your body needs these for optimal health, but it does not produce enough of them, so you must obtain them from food. Foods you will be eating on the 6-Day Fuel Up that are high in PUFAs include cod, halibut, salmon, prawns, tuna, tempeh and tofu. Be aware that not all PUFAs are created equal. Vegetable oils, such as corn, safflower, soybean and sunflower oil, are high in PUFAs but aren't recommended on the Overnight Diet. That's because, when heated, they are easily oxidised, which may have a negative effect on health. You are encouraged to stick to the added fats and fat-free alternatives listed on pages 100–101. (You may be surprised to see butter on that list but the amount you can have is limited and it has the advantage of not containing trans fats – see page 99. If you prefer, you can use a low-calorie spread but make sure it is trans fat free.)

MUFAs are monounsaturated fatty acids. At room temperature, they are typically in liquid form, but when chilled, they become solid. These fats are high in vitamin E, an antioxidant. Foods you will be eating on the 6-Day Fuel Up that are high in MUFAs include avocados, nuts, peanut butter, seeds and olive oil.

If saturated fats are the sticky, gooey stuff that clogs arteries, PUFAs and MUFAs just may be the fats that unclog your arteries so that your blood can flow more freely. Swapping saturated fats for PUFAs and MUFAs results in favourable changes in cholesterol levels that boost protection for your heart.

GET THE LOWDOWN ON THE SCIENCE

PUFA power

A growing body of research has shown that replacing saturated fats with PUFAs decreases the risk of heart disease. Replacing just 1 per cent of saturated fat with PUFAs reduces LDL levels and reduces the risk of coronary events by about 2–3 per cent, according to a 2011 study in the *American Journal of Clinical Nutrition*. In other research, a team of scientists analysed the findings from numerous studies on fat and cardiovascular disease and published their review in the *American Journal of Clinical Nutrition*. They found that for every 5 per cent reduction in intake from saturated fats that was replaced by a concomitant increase in consumption of PUFAs, there was a 10 per cent reduction in the risk of heart disease.

So what about the weight-loss aspect? PUFAs and MUFAs have both been shown to enhance weight loss and decrease the inflammation that has been associated with increased abdominal fat and muscle wasting. MUFA consumption has been linked specifically to reduced abdominal fat. One of the most intriguing studies on MUFAs and body fat appeared in *Diabetes Care* and found that premenopausal women who ate more MUFAs maintained more lean muscle mass than women on a very low-fat diet. In other research from the Czech Republic, obese women lost more weight when consuming more PUFAs.

Just because PUFAs and MUFAs are a better choice than saturated fats, it is still important to remember that all fats are highly caloric. All fats – saturated, PUFA, MUFA – provide 9 calories per gram, and they don't rate high in terms of satiety. In fact, research from a 2010 issue of *Nutrition Journal* revealed that there is no difference in satiety whether you eat saturated fats, PUFAs or MUFAs. Eating PUFAs and MUFAs in the right amount is key. Stick with the portion suggestions in the meal plans and recipes in Chapters 7 and 8 and see the recommendations for added fats below.

Beware of trans fats

One type of fat that can have disastrous effects on your weight and health is trans fats. These fats are used to fry foods like French fries and doughnuts and to help foods like crackers and potato crisps have a longer shelf life. They are also found in margarine. On nutrition labels, you can find them listed as 'partially hydrogenated vegetable oil'. Not only do these fats lead to overall weight gain but they also contribute specifically to abdominal fat, even if you are on a low-calorie diet. Trying to stave off hunger by eating foods like fat-free crackers, cakes and biscuits that are high in trans fats can prevent you from losing the muffin top. Trans fats also raise LDL cholesterol and lower the protective HDL cholesterol, effectively raising the risk of heart disease. There is no place on the Overnight Diet for trans fats. Ditch 'em!

GET THE LOWDOWN ON THE SCIENCE

Trans fats transfer fat to the belly

Researchers at Wake Forest University School of Medicine fed two groups of monkeys a diet that was equal in calories but different in the type of fat consumed. One set of monkeys ate trans fats; the other group ate MUFAs. The

→

number of calories consumed should have maintained their weight without increasing it. But that isn't what happened. The monkeys that ate the trans fats gained 7.2 per cent in body weight compared to 1.8 per cent in the monkeys that ate MUFAs. But what was really troublesome was that the extra fat on the monkeys that ate trans fats all settled in the abdomen. Not only that, fat from other areas of the body migrated to the belly.

Added fats

On the Overnight Diet, you don't have to eliminate added fats, but you will be limiting them to up to 4 servings per day (1 serving = 1 tsp). Focus on healthy added fats that are high in PUFAs and MUFAs, and note that there are many ways to add flavour to dishes without adding fat. Simple ways to do so include using cooking sprays made from olive oil, and fat-free salad dressings and dips. Just these simple switches can dramatically lower your fat consumption and speed you to faster weight loss.

Added fat (you can have up to 4 servings per day; 1 serving = 1 tsp):

Avocado

Low-fat salad dressings

Low-fat dips and sauces

Mayonnaise (made with olive oil)

Butter (or non-trans fat spread)

Olive oil

Nuts

Seeds

Fat-free alternatives:

Cooking sprays (made with olive oil)

Fat-free dips and sauces

Fat-free salad dressings

Prescription no. 4: drink at least 8 glasses of water a day

Staying adequately hydrated while dieting is absolutely essential to keep fat burning in the fast lane. Here are just a couple of the ways being even slightly dehydrated can cause fat burning to slow:

- Dehydration disrupts the metabolism process. Burning calories creates toxins that need to be flushed out of your body. Your kidneys are your body's chief toxin flushers, and they need water to do their job properly. Dehydration reduces their on-the-job performance, creating a backup of toxins in the body. To prevent a potentially dangerous overload of toxins, your kidneys have to call in the liver for back up. But asking your liver to fill in on toxin-flushing duty takes it away from one of its primary functions: metabolising fat. Feed your kidneys water so that your liver can do its job.

- Dehydration robs the body of muscle. Water makes up over 75 per cent of your muscles, and it is critical to the process of building lean muscle. It is also essential for reducing muscle cramps and joint pain, both of which can keep you from doing the physical activities that build lean muscle and boost metabolism. Plus, dehydration reduces blood volume, which lowers the supply of oxygen to your muscles and makes them feel tired. Because maintaining lean muscle is at the foundation of rapid fat burning on this diet, you must keep your muscles adequately hydrated. Hydrated muscle cells are stronger and less likely to be gobbled up for energy.

MYTHBUSTERS

Myth Drinking water will make you retain water and look bloated.

In fact, it's just the opposite. Water retention and the subsequent bloating are signs of dehydration. When your body is deprived of adequate water supplies, it sends off an alert to the brain, which responds by signalling the body's cells to retain water. It's almost as if your body starts building internal dams to keep any water from escaping and, unfortunately, the biggest reservoir of water usually winds up on your abdomen. If you experience abdominal bloating, it could be a sign that you need to drink more fluids.

For adequate hydration, drink at least eight 250ml glasses for a total of 2 litres of water every day. It doesn't matter if you drink tap water, spring water, bottled water or soda water. You can also have flavoured waters, as long as they are unsweetened.

On the Overnight Diet, you can also enjoy black coffee, tea and diet drinks, but these do not count towards your daily requirement of 2 litres of water. In fact, caffeinated beverages are dehydrating, so if you drink 250ml of a caffeinated beverage, you need to offset that by drinking 250ml of water – and that's in addition to the 2 litres.

You can also feel free to enjoy a glass of wine per day – just one however (see opposite)!

GET THE LOWDOWN ON THE SCIENCE

Drink before you eat

To lose weight even faster, drink water before your meals. Research presented at the 2010 National Meeting of the American Chemical Society in Boston found that drinking just two 250ml glasses of water right before you eat increases weight loss. In a trial involving 48 middle-aged and older adults, those who drank water prior to eating consumed an average of 75–90 calories fewer at that meal. The researchers suggest that the water made them feel fuller and less hungry. After 12 weeks, the water drinkers lost more weight compared to those who didn't have water before meals, and they kept the weight off for more than a year. In addition, according to German researchers reporting in the *Journal of Clinical Endocrinology & Metabolism*, within ten minutes of drinking 480ml of water, metabolic rates in both men and women begin to rise and increase by 30 per cent after 30–40 minutes.

What about alcohol?

Research shows that having one alcoholic beverage per day offers health benefits. Wine, as opposed to beer or spirits, gets the stamp of approval on this diet thanks to the many health benefits associated with moderate wine consumption, including:

- Reduced risk of heart disease
- Increased HDL cholesterol
- Reduced risk of type-2 diabetes
- Reduced risk of cancer
- Reduced risk of stroke

- Slowed progression of neurological degenerative disorders like Alzheimer's disease

- Reduced cellular damage from free radicals

- Reduced risk of cataracts

You may have heard that red wine is better than white wine when it comes to heart health, but this may not be true. Both red and white wines have been found to offer protection for your heart. Some research shows that a single glass of wine per day can raise levels of HDL cholesterol, the 'good' cholesterol. So raise a nightly glass of Chardonnay, Cabernet Sauvignon, or Pinot Noir absolutely guilt-free. If you don't drink, don't start. If you do, switch to wine.

Tales of the Measuring Tape

'I've been on lots of diets before that had tiny lists of approved foods. I would get so bored eating the same things over and over, I would have to cheat and go on a binge. Now I get to eat so many of my favourite foods, and I get to drink wine! I never feel like I have to cheat. This is a diet I can live with for the rest of my life.' Jane, 29, dropped 2 stone 3 pounds (14kg) and 6 inches (15cm) off her waist

Putting it all together

On the Overnight Diet, you'll be using these four prescriptions to create delicious, satisfying meals and snacks. Keeping them in mind, the chart below shows an example of what you can eat each day.

_____ minimum weight of protein, according to your DPR	Lean beef, lean pork, poultry, fish, eggs, soya products, meat alternatives, protein powder
Fruit	all you can eat
Non-starchy vegetables	all you can eat
2 servings dairy (1 serving = 240ml)	fat-free or low-fat (1 per cent) yogurt, milk, cottage cheese, dairy alternatives
2–3 servings whole grains (see servings on page 95)	bagel, bread, oatmeal, oat bran, high-fibre cereal, brown rice, brown pasta, crackers, quinoa, couscous
Up to 1 serving starchy veggies/beans, peas and lentils (1 serving = 100g)	sweetcorn, potatoes, squash, sweet potato, black beans, black-eyed beans, cannellini beans, chickpeas, red kidney beans, lentils, butter beans, haricot beans, pinto beans, peas, split peas

chart continues →

Up to 4 servings
added fats
(1 serving = 1 tsp)

avocado, olive oil, low-fat
salad dressings,
mayonnaise, low-fat dips
and sauces, butter (or
non-trans fat spread),
nuts, seeds

Desserts (optional)
(1 serving = as described
in the recipes)

see Meal Plan and
6-Day Fuel Up Recipes
chapters

Wine (optional)
(1 glass = 175ml)

all varieties

Of course, you can get as creative as you like. As you'll see in the 28-Day Meal Plan and 6-Day Fuel Up Recipes chapters, the options are endless.

....

Quickie Rev Up

Did you know that logging endless hours on the treadmill while drastically cutting calories could actually be sabotaging your efforts to lose weight? In addition to making you feel starved and exhausted, it won't help you reach your goal weight. What's the problem? The problem is that this combo of eating less and doing more cardio can put the body into a catabolic state in which it robs the muscles for fuel, effectively slowing metabolism and disrupting the fat-burning process. What should you be doing instead?

As you have already seen, maintaining or developing lean muscle mass is the key to rapid weight loss that lasts while avoiding Shrinking Muscle Syndrome, so your workout needs to focus on increasing lean muscle. But this doesn't mean you have to follow some run-of-the-mill weight-lifting routine. Recent research has revealed that integrating two exercise concepts into one – similar to the way the Overnight Diet combines two diets into one – burns more fat faster than any other workout. It's like getting twice the results in half the time.

GET THE LOWDOWN ON THE SCIENCE

Burn ten times more fat

If you've spent far too much time on the sofa, you might think it's too late for exercise to do your body any good. You'd be wrong! Research in a 2012 issue of *Cell Metabolism* shows that when inactive but otherwise healthy men and women exercise – even for just a few minutes – it results in immediate changes in their DNA. The DNA molecules within the muscles undergo chemical and structural changes that appear to reprogramme the muscles for strength and the metabolic benefits of exercise. This is strong evidence that it is never too late to start exercising and, more importantly, feel the benefits of exercise.

This workout plan relies on a growing body of research showing that combining resistance training with short cardio blasts, called 'Rev Up Blasts' here, into one workout can burn almost ten times more body fat compared to doing strength training and cardio separately. This dynamic approach allows you to strengthen and sculpt your body quickly. The moves are designed specifically to help you tackle those trouble spots, including your tummy, bottom, thighs and batwing arms. And you can get started today, regardless of your age or fitness level. Even better, you don't have to lift a single weight or pound away on the treadmill.

THE BEST KIND OF EXERCISE

Two studies in the *Journal of Strength and Conditioning Research* tested the effectiveness of a traditional workout

→

vs an integrated workout. Here are the two programmes the women participating in the study followed three days a week for 11 weeks:

Group 1: traditional workout	Group 2: integrated workout
Warm-up	Warm-up
Resistance exercises	Alternate between:
Aerobics	high-intensity cardio blast
Cool down	and resistance exercises
	Cool down

The integrated workout produced greater gains in lean muscle, strength, endurance, flexibility and fat-free mass. It also produced a markedly greater decline in fat mass and reduction in body fat percentage. In fact, it produced an almost ten-fold reduction in body fat compared to the group doing the traditional workout.

The Quickie Rev Up burns fat faster

Let's take a look at how this workout will kick fat burning into high gear.

Increases metabolism This workout programme increases lean muscle, and the more lean muscle tissue you have, the higher your basic metabolic rate will be. As you've already seen, a higher metabolism pumps up your body's fat-burning potential throughout the day. Muscle burns seven times more calories than fat. This means that the more lean muscle you have, the more efficient your body will be at burning calories. Classic research from Tufts University and the University of Maryland found that strength training increases basic metabolic rate by 7 per cent and boosts daily calorie expenditure by 15 per cent.

Tales of the Measuring Tape

'I have two toddlers and definitely don't have time to spend an hour a day working out. I needed something that would give me results in a short amount of time. The Quickie Rev Up is the solution. I look more toned than ever, and I love it. I'm wearing tank tops again!' Kristen, 32, lost 1½ stone (9.5kg)

Ramps up the 'after burn' When you alternate between cardio bursts and resistance training moves, you increase something known in scientific circles as excess post-exercise oxygen consumption (EPOC), but which we'll refer to here as the 'after burn'. Basically, the after burn is the number of calories you burn as your body recovers from a workout and returns to a resting state. This means that after you have finished your workout, your body will continue to burn more calories, even while you are watching TV, reading a book or sleeping.

Reduces appetite and food cravings Research shows that strength training can have an almost instantaneous as well as a long-term effect on appetite and those pesky food cravings that threaten to sabotage your weight loss. For several hours following a strength-training session, appetite and cravings decrease. In the long run, building lean muscle through strength training has been found to help balance the appetite hormones, which are often out of whack in overweight and obese people. Cardio alone, on the other hand, does not kill appetite, according to Jim Karas, author of the *New York Times* bestseller *The Cardio-Free Diet*.

Burns more belly fat Interval training, which is similar to the Rev Up cardio blasts you will be doing with the Quickie Rev Up, targets belly fat. It involves alternating between brief bouts of high-intensity activity with periods of lower-intensity exercise, which is exactly what this programme is designed to do. In fact, a team of Australian researchers showed that obese women who did interval training lost three times as much body fat – and significantly more fat from their waistlines – than obese women who performed exercise at a continuous pace.

Reduces insulin resistance As you saw in Chapter 2, Shrinking Muscle Syndrome is associated with insulin resistance, which is a contributing factor in water retention and bloating, both of which make you more likely to have extra padding around your middle. This workout was formulated specifically to help prevent or reverse Shrinking Muscle Syndrome and the insulin resistance that comes with it. The more lean muscle you have, the more effectively your body uses insulin, thereby reducing insulin resistance so that you can eliminate water retention and bloating.

GET THE LOWDOWN ON SCIENCE

Improve your muscle and insulin sensitivity

Research has shown that the components of this workout enhance insulin sensitivity; for example, a report in the *International Journal of Medical Sciences* found that resistance training improves muscle quality and insulin

→

sensitivity in people with type-2 diabetes. In this study, researchers at the University of Maryland tested insulin levels, fat-free mass, body fat percentage and strength in men ages 50–63 both before and after 16 weeks of strength training. At the end of the trial, the men's insulin levels had decreased significantly, signalling an improvement in insulin sensitivity. The drop in insulin was accompanied by a 47 per cent increase in overall strength, a rise in lean tissue and a decrease in body fat percentage. Other research from 2006 in the *Journal of Clinical Endocrinology & Metabolism* also reported that strength training increased insulin sensitivity in obese men.

Interval training has also been found to enhance insulin sensitivity. In one study from 2009 in *BMC Endocrine Disorders*, just two weeks of interval training produced a 23 per cent increase in insulin sensitivity.

Boosts the generation of mitochondria Mitochondria, as outlined previously, are the small powerhouses within your cells that burn food for energy. Evidence shows that exercise causes an upsurge in the numbers of new mitochondria within the cells of your muscles, which enhances muscle vitality, reduces fatigue and improves endurance. Even more exciting is the fact that a small increase in mitochondria reduces the risk of obesity and diabetes. Some research shows that the more muscle groups involved in the exercise you do, the higher the increase in mitochondria. With this exercise programme, you'll be engaging nearly every muscle group in your body.

Increases levels of HGH As you have seen, higher levels of HGH are associated with increases in lean muscle mass and reductions in body fat. The two elements of this hybrid workout have been found to be the ideal combo to naturally boost production of the hormone that has been proven to reduce body fat and increase lean muscle mass. Research in *Mechanisms of Ageing and Development* found that strength training can induce the release of HGH in both the young and elderly, with a greater amount seen in younger people. In 2000, the *Journal of Strength and Conditioning Research* reported a boost in HGH levels in women following a strength-training session, and it didn't matter if the women regularly engaged in strength training or were novices.

The release of HGH following strength training comes as part of the muscle breakdown and regeneration cycle mentioned earlier. As you learned, adequate protein intake is essential to avoid getting stuck in breakdown mode. So is HGH. Strength training causes tiny tears in the muscles and stimulates the production of HGH, which is involved in repairing the muscles.

As a reminder, the Overnight Diet does not suggest that you take HGH supplements to help you achieve your weight-loss goals.

Increases energy levels Physical activity boosts production of AMP-kinase, a metabolic enzyme that provides cellular energy, which puts a little more pep in your step and gives you the energy you need to get off the sofa and move more. AMP-kinase gives you more energy throughout the day and minimises fatigue. Research shows that AMP-kinase is lower in obese people who are insulin resistant compared to obese people who are insulin sensitive.

The Energy Solution

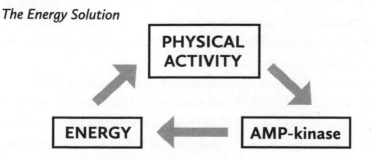

Balances your appetite hormones and fights visceral fat with better sleep Regular exercise has long been associated with improved sleep. In addition to improving your mood during the day, this perk is also something that could be far more beneficial to weight loss than you ever realised. In 2011, the *American Journal of Clinical Nutrition* published a report showing that when you skimp on sleep, you end up eating more. The study involved 15 men and 15 women who slept, in random order, for nine hours a night for five nights and four hours a night for five nights. After getting just four hours of shut-eye for five nights, the study volunteers ate an average of nearly 300 calories more than when they slept for nine hours a night. And those calories came mostly from fat and most notably saturated fat.

Research shows that sleep deprivation wreaks havoc with the body's appetite hormones and leads to visceral fat, the dangerous fat that wraps around your vital organs. In 2010, the National Sleep Foundation in the US reported a 32 per cent increase in visceral fat in people under the age of 40 who slept for fewer than six hours a night.

Other research shows that a shortage of sleep causes a decrease in leptin, the satiety hormone that signals the brain that the body is full, and an increase in ghrelin, the hormone that triggers hunger. The end result is that no matter how much you eat you feel hungry, which makes you more likely to overeat. Getting adequate shut-eye – at least six hours per night – helps balance the appetite hormones, which are primarily produced at night, so it will be easier to control your appetite during the waking hours. And don't think you can just 'catch up' on sleep at weekends. To maintain these benefits, you need to get six or more hours on a consistent basis.

Increases the release of adrenaline to burn stored fat Dr Steven Boutcher is an Australian professor who has carried out groundbreaking research on the kind of short cardio blasts that you'll be doing on this workout. According to Dr Boutcher, these cardio blasts pump up the release of the hormone adrenaline. That's a good thing for weight loss because adrenaline plays a role in breaking down stored fat and burning it. Adrenaline also dampens the appetite, so you'll feel less hungry while you're burning more fat.

Reduces levels of the stress hormone that makes you fat Everybody knows that when you feel stressed you tend to reach for foods that make you fat: chocolate chip cookies, crisps or chips, for example. It's no surprise that people who experience a lot of pressure tend to pack on the pounds. Research shows us that stress and fat feed off each other. When you're under chronic strain, your body releases too much of the stress hormone cortisol, and too much cortisol is what can make you crave and overeat high-fat junk foods. People who are overweight or obese tend to have high levels of cortisol, but so do people who have excess abdominal fat but are slim otherwise. And who wants to have slender arms and legs but a bulging belly? When you exercise on a regular basis, it not only decreases stress but it also improves your resilience to high-pressure situations. And it reduces cortisol levels, which can help you win the battle against stress-eating and stress-related weight gain.

Improves your mood to reduce overeating The mood-boosting benefits of exercise have been well documented, and the proof keeps rolling in; for example, a 2012 study from researchers at Penn State shows that people who get more physical activity tend to feel more excitement and enthusiasm compared to people who are less physically active. These positive feelings may in part be due to the fact that exercise enhances the production of the body's natural feel-good neurochemical endorphins, providing an almost instantaneous mood boost. Not only is this great for your mood but it is also amazing for your waistline. These endorphins also act as an appetite suppressant to help keep eating under control.

Physical activity has also been found to soothe anxiety, relieve low moods and even reduce the incidence of clinical depression, all of which may be triggers for emotional overeating. A growing body of research points to a link between depression and obesity. The good news is that a 2011 review of the scientific evidence on the effect of physical activity on mild depression has found that exercise and physical activity are as effective as antidepressant treatments.

Reduces the risk of injury so that you can stay active When you place stress on your bones through activity, such as strength training, your body responds by reinforcing those bones in a process similar to the breakdown and regeneration of muscle that also occurs with strength training. Having stronger bones makes you less likely to develop osteoporosis or experience bone fractures that can keep you off your feet. Toning your muscles also strengthens the ligaments and tendons that support your joints, reducing your chance of injuries like sprains and strains. When you are injury-free you are more likely to remain active throughout your lifetime!

Improves immune-system function Nothing slows you down like a nasty cold or flu bug. A wealth of scientific research proves that regular exercise shores up your immune system so that you can fight off viruses and infections that might derail your efforts to stay active.

Reduces the risk of chronic disease Decades of research shows that regular exercise reduces your risk of heart disease, stroke, cancer, high blood pressure, diabetes and other debilitating diseases. Regular physical activity strengthens the heart muscle, increases the protective HDL cholesterol, reduces the harmful LDL cholesterol, improves blood flow, reduces blood pressure, improves insulin sensitivity and more. When you aren't sidelined by disease, you are more inclined to remain active.

Why you'll love this workout

Fast fat burning isn't the only benefit you'll enjoy from the Quickie Rev Up. This fun, fast-paced workout strengthens nearly every major muscle group in the body while improving balance and flexibility at the same time. Fun and functional for everyday life, these moves will help you do the things you love to do – chase after your toddler at the park, take your dog for a walk, or play a round of golf – and do them better and more effortlessly! How would you like to run up the stairs without huffing and puffing, or play tennis without feeling destroyed afterwards? Or go dancing without feeling like you're going to slip a disc?

Of course, you want all the benefits that come with regular exercise, but you're busy and don't have hours to dedicate to a workout routine. That's why the Quickie Rev Up has been engineered to provide maximum results in the least amount of time possible. All it takes is 21 minutes four times a week. Out of a total of 10,080 minutes in each week, this routine takes up only 84 of them. Eighty-four out of 10,080 – that's less than 1 per cent of your week! It's a routine that can fit into the craziest hustle-and-bustle lifestyle.

Tales of the Measuring Tape

'I was always afraid that strength training would make me look big and bulky. Boy was I wrong! I'm leaner than ever and my body looks toned but totally feminine. For the first time in my life, I feel confident enough to wear a bikini.'
Caroline, 31, lost 2 stone 9 pounds (16.7kg)

The Quickie Rev Up won't leave you yawning from boredom either. With ten different strength-training moves to choose from and ten different ways to do the Rev Up Blasts, this routine keeps you and your muscles guessing, to prevent the fitness plateaus that occur when doing the same exercises over and over. After all, your body is incredibly smart. It adapts quickly to exercise, becoming so efficient at the various moves that it takes less and less effort to perform them.

When you first start the programme, you may find some of the moves challenging. But after just a few weeks, your body will adapt to them and you will find that they seem easier and that you are ready to pump up the intensity. This is progress! But your body is so good at adapting that if you do the same moves over and over and over, you may stop seeing that progress. To avoid such plateaus, you need to switch your workout routine. Changing a couple of the moves you do, or doing them in a different order, may be all it takes to keep challenging your muscles so that you keep getting leaner and more toned.

Rest assured, this workout can be tailored for all fitness levels. If you're a complete novice, you don't need to feel intimidated, because the moves can be modified to make them easier. And you can rev up the intensity as you progress.

Tales of the Measuring Tape

'I thought I was too fat to exercise, but the Quickie Rev Up offered ways to make each of the moves easier. So I just did the easier options at first and that gave me the confidence I needed to keep going. Now I'm doing the more advanced options, which I never would have imagined I could do. I look and feel like a completely different person.'
Alberto, 51, lost 7 stone 11 pounds (49.4kg)

One of the best things about the Quickie Rev Up is that it requires almost nothing besides your body. You don't have to join a fancy, expensive gym or invest in a lot of pricey equipment. You can do it anytime, anywhere: in your own home, at a park or in a hotel room if you're travelling. Of course, if you enjoy working out with weights or you like the idea of going to a gym, you'll see how to do the exercises with weights or machines too. The choice is up to you. The illustrations will show you exactly how to do each move.

MYTHBUSTERS

Myth Strength training makes women bulk up and look manly.

If you're afraid that strength training is going to make you look like the Incredible Hulk, stop your fretting. Rest assured, the Quickie Rev Up is not designed to make you bulk up like a hard-core bodybuilder. It's designed, first and foremost, to help you maintain the muscle you already have so that you can avoid Shrinking Muscle Syndrome. Any increases in lean tissue will simply give you a more toned, fit appearance. Bulking up typically results from a combination of several contributing factors, including lifting heavy weights (which you won't be doing), dedicating several hours a day to weight training (which you won't be doing), the hormone testosterone (which women do not produce in sufficient quantities to increase muscle size) and a caloric surplus (which you won't have on this diet).

Important! Check with your doctor before starting any exercise programme.

Quickie Rev Up basics

The workout starts with a dynamic warm-up, which then alternates between strength-training moves and 60-second Rev Up Blasts. It is most important to keep it quick! It is called the Quickie Rev Up for three reasons. First, the whole thing takes just 21 minutes. Second, it is engineered to reshape your body quickly. And third, it is important that you go from move to move quickly without taking any breaks. As soon as you complete the dynamic warm-up, jump right into your first strength-training move then into your first Rev Up Blast and back to the next strength-training move. It'll be over before you know it. Now let's break it down.

Dynamic warm-up

Forget about the static stretching your school gym teacher might have had you do as a 'warm-up' before gym class. Emerging research shows that this type of old-school stretching actually reduces performance and may even increase the risk of injury, while a dynamic warm-up boosts your athletic abilities and helps prevent sprains and muscle strains. In fact, according to Australian researcher James Zois, at the School of Sport and Exercise Science at Victoria University in Melbourne, there is an 11 per cent difference in performance depending on whether you do static stretching or a dynamic warm-up before physical activity – with the dynamic warm-up coming out on top.

This do-anywhere first step prepares your body to crank up your performance for even faster results while minimising the risk of injury. It consists of five simple moves that you will do in rapid succession for a total of three minutes, but we'll get into the specifics in Chapter 9. In just those three minutes, this warm-up will:

- Activate your muscles from head to toe.
- Warm up your muscles and ligaments to prevent injury.

- Open up your joints to improve mobility.

- Wake up your nervous system to help your body coordinate your movement.

- Increase blood flow to send more oxygen to the muscles.

The dynamic warm-up is essential in helping you get the most out of the Quickie Rev Up, so don't skip it.

Strength-training moves

As we've discussed, strength training is absolutely essential for maintaining lean muscle mass and preventing Shrinking Muscle Syndrome. Starting at age 25, adults who don't strength train lose an average of at least half a pound (225g) of lean muscle tissue each year. It is estimated that people lose 30 per cent of their muscle strength between the ages of 50 and 70.

The only way to develop lean muscle mass is to expose the muscles to some form of resistance, such as your own body weight, free weights or machines. During strength training, which may also be referred to as resistance training, muscle fibres are broken down and then quickly repaired by the body. Remember when we discussed your body being like a factory? After strength training, your factory workers rush in to mend the torn or injured muscle fibres, and they throw in some extra padding (aka more fibres) while they're at it to help shore up those muscles. It is this ongoing cycle of breakdown and repair that preserves and builds lean muscle.

Most people are surprised to discover that it isn't the strength training that actually makes muscles get bigger. Rather, it's the repair process that is set in motion to heal the tiny 'injuries' to the muscles caused by resistance training that ultimately strengthens them and increases their size. The repair process starts taking place almost immediately after you complete a resistance-training workout.

The body-weight moves in this programme are designed to provide the resistance you need to break down muscle tissue and stimulate the repair process. They incorporate several muscle groups at once so you get more results in less time. There are five Quickie Rev Up Foundation Moves and ten Quickie Rev Up Advanced Moves. The first are called Foundation Moves because they provide the foundation for the more advanced exercises. This is why it is critical that you learn them first. Regardless of your current fitness level, it is recommended that you spend at least two weeks doing the five Foundation Moves before tackling the Advanced Moves. But don't feel pressured to progress to the Advanced Moves. The Foundation Moves work nearly every muscle in your body, so if they continue to provide enough challenge for you week after week, stick with them! Along with the basics of each move, you'll find tips on how to make it easier or how to increase the intensity, depending on your fitness level.

In Chapter 9, you will find illustrations and easy-to-follow step-by-step instructions for each of the body-weight moves customised for all fitness levels. You can mix and match with simple routines that alternate in order to continually challenge the muscles, which will prevent them – and you – from becoming bored. Even if you are doing the five Quickie Rev Up Foundation Moves, you should change the order in which you do them to prevent boredom.

MYTHBUSTERS

Myth Strength training makes your muscles so sore, you can barely move the next day.

If you wake up the morning after doing your Quickie Rev Up routine and feel like you've been run over by a truck, you've

→

probably overdone it and should scale back the intensity of your workout. Strength training at the appropriate intensity will probably cause mild muscle soreness the following day, or rather 'muscle awareness'. This means that you are aware of the muscles you worked and you can tell that you challenged them, but they are not aching. If you are very sore, take a day off to rest your muscles before exercising again. If soreness is due to an injury, check with your doctor before exercising.

Rev Up Blasts

These cardio blasts will get your heart pumping and fire up fat burning by depleting the glycogen stores in your muscles. They will also boost your cardiovascular endurance and give you that feel-good endorphin rush. The best part is they only take 60 seconds. You don't have to jog for an hour on the treadmill, spend 45 minutes climbing on the stair climber or force yourself to do 30 minutes on the elliptical machine. You go as hard as you can for 60 seconds. To get the most bang for your buck from the Rev Up Blasts, you really have to give it your all. You can do anything for 60 seconds, right?

The Quickie Rev Up provides ten simple ways to do the 60-second Rev Up Blasts, including speed walking and jogging in place. Again these don't require any equipment, so you can do them anywhere, anytime. The most important thing to remember is that it's quickly jumping from the strength-training moves to the Rev Up Blasts and back again that works magic on your muscles and fires up metabolism. Don't skip one or the other. As with the combination of the 1-Day Power Up and the 6-Day Fuel Up, it's the combination of the strength-training moves and Rev Up Blasts that make this workout the fastest fat burner you can find.

SAMPLE QUICKIE REV UP WORKOUT

- Dynamic warm-up   3 minutes
- Strength-training move   3 minutes
- Rev Up Blast   1 minute
- Strength-training move   3 minutes
- Strength-training move   3 minutes
- Rev Up Blast   1 minute
- Strength-training move   3 minutes
- Strength-training move   3 minutes
- Rev Up Blast   1 minute

What should you eat and drink before and after the Quickie Rev Up?

As a general rule, the energy you use during exercise doesn't come from the food you put into your body immediately prior to working out. It's the glycogen stored in your muscles and fat cells that fuel your workout. With the Overnight Diet, you will be filling up on foods that fuel your muscles and boost your energy and you will be staying adequately hydrated. This means you don't need to stress about pre-workout snacks.

What about after your workout? That's a different story. As you recall, strength training breaks down muscle tissue. To put a halt to that breakdown process and to fuel the recovery and repair process that rebuilds and grows your muscles, you need protein; protein is the building block of muscle, after all. Ideally, you should eat something that contains lean protein within half an hour of completing the Quickie Rev Up. Doing so will help stimulate the repair process that will give you the long, lean, toned muscles you want. That glycogen in your muscles you just spent on your workout needs to be replaced as well. On the Overnight Diet, fruit and vegetables along with whole grains do the trick. If you don't have time for a full meal, try a protein-filled snack with healthy carbs to promote the repair and replenish process. Here are a few good examples:

- Fat-free Greek yogurt with berries
- Natural, fat-free yogurt with a spoonful of protein powder and an apple
- Low-fat cottage cheese with pineapple pieces
- Half a turkey sandwich on wholemeal bread
- 1 medium apple with 1 tsp peanut butter
- 1 hard-boiled egg and 1 slice of wholemeal toast

On the days you do the Quickie Rev Up, it is a good idea to drink at least 250ml of water prior to starting your workout, another 250ml of water while you workout, and 250ml more after you finish to aid the recovery process. If you sweat excessively or it is extremely hot or humid, you may need even more fluids.

Quickie Rev Up fitness assessment

Whether you have never broken into a sweat in your entire life or you are a regular exerciser, the Quickie Rev Up can be tailored to suit your individual needs. It is important to work at the appropriate level to prevent injury and to help you stay motivated so that you can get the maximum fat-burning effect. Trying an advanced routine when you are a beginner can be demoralising and make you want to throw in the towel. But when you work out at the appropriate level for you, you will see progress quickly and be able to enjoy a slimmer, trimmer, more toned body faster than you ever thought possible. Answer the following questions to find your fitness level so that you can get the most out of your Quickie Rev Up.

Questionnaire

1. *What is your age?*

    a. Over 50
    b. 30–49
    c. Under 30

2. *What is your BMI?*

    a. Over 35
    b. 30–35
    c. Under 30

3. *How often are you physically active?*

    a. I don't engage in any physical activity.
    b. I participate in physical activity occasionally (less than three times per week).
    c. I am physically active on a regular basis (at least three times per week).

4. *Do you strength train?*

    a. I have never done strength training.
    b. I have done strength training but do not do it on a regular basis (less than twice a week).
    c. I do strength training regularly (at least twice a week).

5. *Which best describes your ability to do a push-up?*

    a. I can't do any kind of push-up.
    b. I can do at least one push-up with my knees touching the ground.
    c. I can do at least one traditional push-up.

6. *How much cardio endurance do you have?*

    a. I get tired moving from the sofa to the fridge.
    b. I can walk briskly for 5–15 minutes before getting tired.
    c. I can walk briskly for more than 15 minutes without getting tired.

7. *Which best describes your flexibility?*

    a. I don't even come close to touching my toes when I bend over.
    b. When I bend over, my fingertips are within a couple of inches of my toes.
    c. I can put my fingertips or whole hands on the floor when I bend over.

8. *Do you have any chronic aches or pains (back, knees, hips, feet, etc.)?*

    a. I am in constant pain.
    b. I have some issues with pain but not all the time.
    c. I do not have chronic pain.

Score

Mostly As: Make it Easier

You're new to fitness or it's been a while since you've broken into a sweat, and you may have some issues with pain that have kept you on the sidelines. Use the 'Make it Easier' options for the five Quickie Rev Up Foundation Moves for at least two weeks or until you get the hang of the exercises and build up your confidence, strength and endurance. When you feel comfortable with the 'Make it Easier' versions, you can step up to the basic versions and pat yourself on the back for a job well done.

Mostly Bs: Basic Move

You may be like so many busy people who sporadically squeeze in a workout here and there. Or perhaps you are one of those people who go through phases – working out like crazy for a few months and then dropping it altogether. Developing consistency is key to igniting the breakdown and repair processes that increase lean muscle mass to keep fat burning in the fast lane. Start with the 'Basic Move' options of the five Quickie Rev Up Foundation Moves for at least two full weeks before advancing to the 'Rev It Up' options.

Mostly Cs: Rev It Up

You engage in some form of exercise on a regular basis and are probably raring to take advantage of the fat-burning potential of the Quickie Rev Up. Start with the 'Rev It Up' versions of the five Quickie Rev Up Foundation Moves for the first two weeks before progressing to the Quickie Rev Up Advanced Moves. It is important that you master the proper form and technique of these moves to see maximum fat-burning results.

You will find the exercise routine and helpful illustrations in Chapter 9.

PART 3

....

The Overnight Diet Made Easy

....

CHAPTER SIX

28-Day Meal Plan

On most diets, you have to starve yourself into your skinny jeans. Not on this one. When you look at the following 28-day meal plan, you'll be amazed by how much food – and how many kinds of foods – you get to eat. You'll even be enjoying pizza, chilli, burgers and cheesecake – all while burning fat and losing weight. It's time for you to say goodbye to hunger and deprivation and hello to a delicious bounty of satisfying food.

How to use Chapter 6

The 28-day meal plan offers an easy-to-follow blueprint. The 1-Day Power Up days, which fall on Day 1 of each week, are a cinch: three delicious, satisfying, jumbo smoothies that will torch fat while keeping hunger at bay. On the 6-Day Fuel Up days, you'll be eating breakfast, lunch and dinner, plus three snacks a day (optional) and dessert (optional). The 6-Day Fuel Up days have been created with the four prescriptions from Chapter 4 in mind:

- **Prescription no. 1: meet your DPR every day** Remember your daily total quantity of lean meat, fish or poultry, or your vegetarian alternative.

- **Prescription no. 2: stick to lean carbs** Enjoy your all-you-can-eat fruits and non-starchy vegetables, eat up to 100g of starchy veggies, and 2–3 servings of whole grains (see page 95) absolutely guilt-free.

- **Prescription no. 3: focus on healthy fats,** but remember it is possible to have too much of a good thing – so only eat up to 4 servings daily (see page 100).

- **Prescription no. 4: drink at least 8 glasses of water a day**, and feel free to enjoy one glass of wine.

> **Important!** Adjust the protein quantities to meet your DPR.

The daily meal plans here have been designed for someone with a DPR of 400g of protein (that's total protein foods in the form of lean meat, fish, poultry, eggs or high-protein vegetarian sources) per day on the 6-Day Fuel Up. Referring back to the chart in Chapter 4, women who have an ideal weight of about 10–10 stone 9 pounds (63.5–67.6kg) and men with an ideal weight of about 10 stone 2 pounds–10 stone 13 pounds (54.4–69kg) have a DPR that works out at 400g. Depending on your individual DPR, you will need to adjust the amount of protein in the daily meal plans to meet your needs.

Remember, the protein sources that count towards your DPR for the 6-Day Fuel Up are:

- Lean beef
- Lean pork
- Fish
- Poultry
- Eggs

- Soya products and meat alternatives
- Protein powder

It is imperative that you adjust the quantities of these specific protein sources in this meal plan and in the recipes to meet your individual minimum DPR. To make it easier for you, the recipes in Chapter 8 indicate the protein sources you need to adjust. But note that there is no need to adjust any other ingredients or serving sizes.

Here's how to do it: the meal plan is designed to provide 400g of protein food a day: 60g at breakfast, 115g at lunch and 225g at dinner. When adjusting recipes for your DPR, the simplest thing to do is look at the day's meals that specify protein in grams – say, 115g of salmon as on Week 1, Day 5 on page 146 – and add or subtract what you need. If your DPR is 375g per day, you would subtract 25g and have 90g of salmon. If your DPR is 425g, you would add 25g and have 140g. All of the other meals on that day would stay the same. That's the only adjustment you would need to make.

What if the day's plan – like Week 1, Day 2 on page 141 – is made up of meals like Spicy Chicken and Cannellini Bean Chilli, which serves 4, and Crusty Oven-fried Fish, which also serves 4? Again, it's simple. At the top of each recipe in Chapter 8, you'll see 'Protein per serving towards DPR', which shows you the total amount of protein in each serving. You can either adjust both lunch and dinner to meet your needs or modify only one of those meals and leave the rest of the day's meals the same – whatever is simplest for you. (Note: it is generally easier to adjust lunches and dinners – rather than breakfast – as these are the biggest sources of protein.) Remember, it's your daily protein total that is most important.

To illustrate this adjustment, let's look at how two different people, both with unique DPRs, would make adjustments for Week 1, Day 5 (115g salmon for lunch) and Week 1, Day 2 (1 serving Spicy Chicken and Cannellini Bean Chilli for lunch and 1 serving Crusty Oven-fried Fish for dinner).

Kim's ideal weight is 7 stone 12 pounds (49.9kg), so her DPR is 350g per day, because, if you remember, 350g is the minimum DPR for all adults, regardless of your ideal weight. And since your DPR is the *minimum* amount of protein you should be consuming, Kim isn't required to decrease the amount of protein in the daily meal plans (as they provide 400g of protein per day). But if she wants to, she can reduce the daily meal plans by 50g of protein per day. So how would she do that?

Week 1, Day 5: instead of 115g of salmon at lunch, Kim would have 65g of salmon and the rest of the day's meals would remain the same.

Week 1, Day 2: to eliminate 50g of protein, Kim could reduce lunch and dinner by 25g each or simply reduce dinner by 50g. Here's how. The chilli recipe calls for 460g of chicken breast for 4 servings, which means there are 115g of chicken in each serving. Reducing each serving by 25g means she would need 90g of chicken per serving, or a total of 360g to make 4 servings. The fish recipe calls for 4 × 225g pieces of cod. Simply adjust that to 4 pieces that are 200g each. This way, Kim has eliminated 25g from lunch and 25g from dinner. She could also keep one of the recipes as it is, say the chilli recipe, and modify only the fish recipe, reducing each serving by 50g so that she would use 4 × 175g pieces of cod. There is no need to alter any other ingredient amounts in the recipes.

Mark's ideal weight is 13 stone 2 pounds (83.4kg), so his DPR is 500g of protein per day. He needs to add 100g of protein per day to the daily meal plans.

Week 1, Day 5: instead of 115g of salmon at lunch, Mark would have 215g of salmon, and the rest of the day's meals would remain the same.

Week 1, Day 2: to add 100g of protein, he could add 50g to each of lunch and dinner or simply add 100g to dinner. Here's how. The chilli recipe calls for 460g of chicken for 4 servings, which means there are 115g of chicken in each serving. Increasing each serving by 50g means he would need 165g of chicken per serving, or a total of 660g of chicken to make 4 servings. The fish recipe calls for 4 × 225g pieces of cod. Simply adjust that to 4 pieces that are 275g each. This way, Mark has added 50g to lunch and 50g to dinner. He could also keep one of the recipes as it is, say the chilli recipe, and modify the fish recipe, increasing each serving by 100g, so he would use 4 × 325g pieces of cod. There is no need to alter any other ingredient amounts in the recipes.

CALCULATING EGGS AND VEGETARIAN SOURCES OF PROTEIN

When calculating your protein for the day, bear in mind that eggs and vegetarian sources of protein need to be calculated using the chart on page 88, because, unlike meat and fish, the weight of the product does not directly correlate to the contribution towards your total DPR. (The only exception is seitan.) In the case of tofu, for example, you would need to eat 85g in order to gain 30g towards your *total* DPR for the day. See pages 87–8 for further guidance.

Meal plan dos and don'ts

- Do start with the 1-Day Power Up on Day 1 and each week thereafter.

- Do follow the four prescriptions for the 6-Day Fuel Up on days 2–7 of each week.

- Don't skip any meals (it's OK to skip snacks and dessert; they're optional), or you won't be getting adequate protein.

- Don't combine meals, for example eating lunch and dinner all together in one huge meal. The body can only process so much protein at one time.

Take advantage of flexibility

Flexibility is an integral part of this programme, so even though smoothies, meals and snacks are clearly outlined, feel free to make substitutions within the parameters of the diet; for example, the three smoothies listed for Day 1 of each week have been selected to spark weight loss and ensure a variety of flavours. But Chapter 7 will give you more details on how to select three smoothies of your choosing for your 1-Day Power Up. You can also replace any of the suggested smoothies with one of your own creation using the Mix 'n' Match Smoothie Chart on page 346. You'll find more on this in Chapter 7 too.

The 6-Day Fuel Up recommendations are also interchangeable. If you don't eat pork, it's OK to have chicken, beef, fish or soya products instead. If you aren't a fan of broccoli, but you do like spinach, then by all means have spinach. If you prefer brown rice to couscous, go with the whole grain you prefer. Just be sure when making these types of substitutions that you use the correct quantities given on page 95: for example, if the meal plan calls for 80g of couscous, cooked (or 30g uncooked) – as 1 serving – then swap it for 1 serving of brown rice (80g, cooked or 30g uncooked), and so on. Quantities for the vegetable accompaniments are not given where these are from the all-you-can-eat list but make sure you have plenty of these healthy vegetables, they'll help fill you up. And remember, coffee, tea, in-between meal snacks, dessert and a nightly glass of wine are all optional.

As well as featuring the recipes from the menu plan, Chapter 8 has some other favourite recipes that you may enjoy, but please bear in mind that where recipes do not specify a DPR you must accompany them with a source of protein when serving them as part of a main meal.

Meal timing

Your meal timing is also flexible. One question that is asked a lot is: 'How long do I wait in between meals and snacks?' Generally, it's a good idea to space out meals and snacks every two to three hours. Here's how this might look:

8.00am – breakfast

10.30am – snack

1.00pm – lunch

3.30pm – snack

6.00pm – dinner and dessert

8.30pm – snack

Sticking to this type of schedule is advisable because it helps prevent hunger throughout the day. Of course, with a hectic lifestyle, it is not always possible. You might have a crazy day at work and not get round to eating lunch until three o'clock. You might have to shuttle the kids from school to football to a play date and miss your afternoon snack. Or you might be a student who keeps funny hours and ends up eating dinner at 11.00pm. That's what happened to Melinda, a patient at the Nutrition and Weight Management Center at Boston Medical Center who was studying at medical school.

....

CASE STUDY *Melinda*

Melinda had tutorials all day long then spent long hours studying at the library and sometimes wouldn't get round to dinner until late at night. That's OK. Occasionally moving off the schedule won't disrupt the metabolic improvements provided by the Overnight Diet; however, if you find that you are regularly off schedule, be sure to keep fruits and veggies to hand for snacking to tide you over until you have a chance to eat your meal.

....

Shopping guide

Having all the ingredients you need for the week's meals and smoothies to hand helps ensure your weight-loss success. To make sure you're prepared for the coming week, take time on your 1-Day Power Up to review the entire week of menus and make shopping lists (consult the Overnight Diet Shopping List on page 349) for when you go shopping. If you see that some of the week's recipes are best made a day or two in advance, consider preparing them on your rest and relaxation day. Look for these and other time-saving tips in the Time Saver boxes throughout this chapter.

As you'll notice, many of the meals in this plan call for fat-free, low-fat or high-protein foods. What exactly do I mean by that? Here is what to look for when shopping for these products:

- High-fibre cereals: at least 6g of fibre per 100g (and sugar-free).

- Sugar-free: less than 0.5g of sugar per serving. Contains no ingredient that is sugar. Look for 'No Added Sugar' and 'Without Added Sugar' labels.

- Low-sugar yogurt: 12g of sugar or less.

- Fat-free: less than 0.5g of fat per serving. Contains no ingredient that is a fat.

- Low-fat (1 per cent): 3g of fat or less.

- Low-salt: less than 140mg sodium per serving.

- No-salt: less than 5mg sodium per serving.

Do bear in mind that the precise guidelines as to what can be called 'low-fat', 'low-salt' and so on vary from country to country, therefore you need to examine the nutritional label – and not simply trust the flash on the front – to ensure that they conform to the levels we're aiming for with this diet.

SOURCING FAT-FREE INGREDIENTS

Fat-free versions of everyday foods are a good way of adding flavour to your diet – without all the fat and calories that standard products contain – and more and more of these products are becoming available in supermarkets. The following products are particularly useful and although not widely available in all supermarkets, are worth sourcing:

Fat-free chocolate syrup is a great way to add a chocolate flavour, particularly to smoothies. If you can't find it at your local supermarket try online retailers specialising in sweets and candy from the US.

Fat-free salsa is very useful as an accompaniment to crudités and for adding extra flavour to main courses. As tomato is the main ingredient it should be relatively easy to find a fat-free version – be warned though, often those from the deli counter include fat, while the cheaper, jarred versions are more likely to be fat free. You'll find a few fat-free salsa recipes in the 'Dips' section.

Fat-free dips, other than salsa, can be very difficult to find, as dips are often loaded with fat. Look out for yogurt and cucumber dips and salsas made with fruit. Alternatively, make your own – you'll find a number of delicious recipes in the 'Dips' section.

Fat-free frozen yogurt can now be found in a number of large supermarkets, albeit in a limited range of flavours. If you have a favourite fat-free yogurt flavour that isn't available frozen, why not freeze it yourself and enjoy it as a dessert.

Benefit from all-you-can-eat fruit and non-starchy veg

The fruit and non-starchy veggies that are included in your all-you-can-eat list (see page 350–3) can replace any of the snack suggestions and is something you can turn to when you feel hungry. Always have some fresh fruits and veggies ready-prepared and to hand for these times. Also make individual snack bags of veggies so that you can just grab them and go in the morning.

And why not treat yourself to a spa beverage?

On pages 281–7 you'll find a selection of healthy, low-calorie drinks for you to enjoy – so you won't feel deprived of those naughtier drinks that can derail your weight-loss efforts. These drinks are good enough for you to imagine you're spoiling yourself at a health spa!

Week 1, Day 1

1-Day Power Up

Welcome to your first 1-Day Power Up. You may be feeling a bit unsure about what to expect, but just take a look at these enticing, mouth-watering, jumbo smoothies. Each recipe will fill you up and prime your body to burn more fat all day – and all night – long. So cast aside any sense of hesitation and dive right in to rev up rapid weight loss.

BREAKFAST
Banana Latte Smoothie, page 176

Kickstart your day with a smoothie so delicious it belongs on the menu of your favourite coffee house.

LUNCH
Orange Zest Smoothie, page 179

This zesty citrus explosion is like sunshine in a blender – who knew a smoothie lunch could taste so sinfully delicious?

DINNER
Green Apple Goddess Smoothie, page 182

Tangy bits of green apple dotted with hints of sweetness fill you up completely. No hunger here as you complete your first 1-Day Power Up.

HERE'S THE LOWDOWN

Be generous with the veggies in your smoothies. You won't even taste them, and their high-fibre content bulks up the volume so you will feel full faster and stay that way longer.

TIME SAVER

Consider making tomorrow's Spicy Chicken and Cannellini Bean Chilli and the following day's Hot Black-Eyed Bean Soup today. Chilli and soup usually taste better after the flavours have had a chance to blend. Make extra and freeze in pre-portioned storage containers for quick and easy meals at a later date.

Week 1, Day 2

6-Day Fuel Up

BREAKFAST
Grapefruit segments
250g fat-free Greek yogurt
Crustless Quiche, page 192
½ wholemeal bagel
Coffee or tea with skimmed milk and Truvia or Splenda

SNACK
Baby carrots with Savoury Yogurt Dip, page 264

LUNCH
Spicy Chicken and Cannellini Bean Chilli, page 230
Salad with baby spinach, mandarin orange slices, 1 tbsp slivered
   almonds, fat-free dressing
80g cooked brown rice

SNACK
Grapes

DINNER
Crusty Oven-fried Fish, page 241
Roasted Garlic Cauliflower Mash, page 256
Green beans, cooked

DESSERT
100ml (2 small scoops) fat-free frozen yogurt
1 low-fat gingernut biscuit

SNACK
Blueberries and pineapple chunks

HERE'S THE LOWDOWN

How do you eat just one biscuit or chocolate chip cookie? If you buy an entire packet and nibble on just one of them, then you have to try to ignore the tempting siren call of the rest of those tasty treats in the cupboard, and you know how impossible that is. Having junk food or treats in the house is one of the most common reasons why people fall off a healthy eating plan. It's best to keep trigger foods out of your kitchen. If you want a treat, buy one small cookie from your supermarket bakery (or share one if they only do large sizes). Don't buy a whole packet – even though they're cheaper that way – and try to convince yourself that you will have the willpower to eat just one of them. You won't.

Enlist the help of friends and family for situations like these. Here are a few tricks:

- Split the cost of a packet with a friend, take one biscuit, and give the rest of the packet to your friend. Ask her to dole them out to you according to a pre-approved schedule.

- Buy a packet, take one biscuit, and ask your spouse to take the rest of them to his or her place of work.

- If you like home-made biscuits or cookies, make a small amount of dough, divide it into individual portions and store it in the freezer. When it's your 'cookie' night, take one out, bake it, and savour the freshly baked flavour.

- Go for a low-calorie snack pack. You'll get the satisfaction of eating more than one, but because they are so small, they won't do a lot of damage.

Week 1, Day 3

6-Day Fuel Up

BREAKFAST
40–50g high-fibre cereal
Fresh berries
200ml skimmed milk
250g fat-free Greek yogurt mixed with ⅔ scoop protein powder
Coffee or tea with skimmed milk and Truvia or Splenda

SNACK
Kiwi fruit and strawberry slices

LUNCH
Hot Black-Eyed Bean and Chicken Soup, page 210
Steamed broccoli with lemon

SNACK
Apple wedges with fat-free dip

DINNER
225g gammon steak, pan-fried in a non-stick pan with olive
    oil spray
Swiss chard with garlic and parsley, stir-fried
Rice Pilaff, page 257

DESSERT
Chocolate brownie, 5cm square
100ml (2 small scoops) fat-free frozen yogurt

SNACK
Thawed frozen or fresh peaches

TIME SAVER

Soak the red kidney beans today for tomorrow's Bean, Corn
and Quinoa Salad. Rinse and drain the soaked beans and
add fresh water for cooking to reduce the gas that beans
can cause. Tease out some 'me time' later in the week by
cooking extra beans today for breakfast on Week 1, Day
5 and dinner on Week 1, Day 7. Chill in the fridge until
needed. Or, simply can it! When you're short of time, opt
for canned beans rather than dried beans. You'll get all the
flavour and all the health benefits without all that prep time
needed to soak and cook dried beans.

Week 1, Day 4

6-Day Fuel Up

BREAKFAST
½ grapefruit, lightly toasted under the grill
Egg and Spinach Omelette, page 195
1 thin slice wholemeal toast
Coffee or tea with skimmed milk and Truvia or Splenda

SNACK
Sliced pear with fat-free dip

LUNCH
Bean, Corn and Quinoa Salad, page 248
115g pan-fried mini chicken fillets
Carrot slices, cooked

SNACK
Thawed frozen or fresh mango

DINNER

225g pan-seared wild salmon (liberally sprinkle with freshly
ground black pepper before cooking)
Avocado, Fennel and Citrus Salad, page 250
Baby spinach, stir-fried with olive oil spray

DESSERT

250g fat-free yogurt
1 chocolate chip cookie, 5cm diameter

SNACK

One small handful of mixed dried cranberries and raisins
(see box below)

TIME SAVER

Get a jump on tomorrow: cook an extra 115g of salmon
fillet tonight for tomorrow's lunch. (Cook the salmon for 4
minutes on each side or until cooked through.)

HERE'S THE LOWDOWN

Dried fruit is created by removing most of the water
content from the fresh fruit. Dried fruit retains most of its
nutritional content and dietary fibre, but the pack varieties
sold on store shelves are often infused with some form of
sugar to add sweetness, and they are more energy dense
than their fresh fruit counterparts; for example, a large
handful of fresh grapes has 104 calories, but a large handful
of raisins packs 434 calories. Because of this, you should
limit dried fruits to no more than one small handful a day.

Week 1, Day 5

6-Day Fuel Up

BREAKFAST
1 orange
Poached Eggs with Beans, page 191
Coffee or tea with skimmed milk and Truvia or Splenda

SNACK
Baked Cinnamon Apples, page 259

LUNCH
115g pan-seared wild salmon
Oven-roasted cauliflower with olive oil and black pepper
1 small serving Spicy Peanut Noodles, page 217

SNACK
Pineapple slices

DINNER
Pork Escalopes with Caribbean Salsa, page 238
Green beans, steamed
Broccoli, steamed

DESSERT
1 serving Smart Brownies, page 277
1 tbsp low-fat crème fraîche

SNACK
Grapes

Week 1, Day 6

6-Day Fuel Up

BREAKFAST
1 orange
250g fat-free yogurt
1 slice turkey rasher
1 egg, poached
½ wholemeal bagel or 1 thin slice wholemeal toast
Coffee or tea with skimmed milk and Truvia or Splenda

SNACK
Star fruit or kiwi fruit

LUNCH
Beefy Mushroom Burger, page 233
Side salad with fat-free dressing
250ml skimmed milk

SNACK
Cherries

DINNER
Zesty Broccoli Coleslaw Salad with Chicken, page 229

DESSERT
Apple and Cranberry Crumble, page 272

SNACK
Carrot and celery sticks

Week 1, Day 7

6-Day Fuel Up

BREAKFAST
1 sliced banana
250g fat-free yogurt
2 poached eggs
1 thin slice wholemeal toast
Coffee or tea with skimmed milk and Truvia or Splenda

SNACK
Frozen mixed fruit

LUNCH
Spicy 'Pepperoni' Pizza, page 216
Mixed salad leaves, tomatoes, cucumber, red onion slices, 1 tbsp
  fat-free Italian salad dressing

SNACK
Blueberries

DINNER
Red Kidney Bean and Chicken Chilli, page 220
Baby spinach and garlic, stir-fried

DESSERT
Peachy Oat Crumble, page 275

SNACK
1 apple

TIME SAVER

Say hello to a quick and easy day! Use the reserved red kidney beans from Week 1, Day 4 and use a wholemeal pizza crust for a fast and easy pizza lunch.

Week 2, Day 1

1-Day Power Up

Congratulations – you've already completed your first week! By now, the number on your scales is going down and you're motivated to keep it heading in that direction. Your second smoothie day will stoke your body's fat-burning engines.

BREAKFAST
Crispy Apple Smoothie, page 181

Wake up to a crispy apple smoothie teeming with juicy bursts of citrus! Protein powder, fruits and veggies guarantee boundless energy and enthusiasm to get your day off to a great start.

LUNCH
Chocolate Banana Swirl Smoothie, page 180

Scents of cinnamon and chocolate in your glass to delight the senses and provide total satisfaction.

DINNER
Green Machine Smoothie, page 178

End your day with a savoury smoothie that's voluminous in flavour and fullness.

TIME SAVER

Make Overnight Power Oats, page 198, today for tomorrow's breakfast.

Week 2, Day 2

6-Day Fuel Up

BREAKFAST
Overnight Power Oats, page 198
Coffee or tea with skimmed milk and Truvia or Splenda

SNACK
Stewed eating apples with cinnamon

LUNCH
Tuna wrap sandwich made with:
Mediterranean Tuna Salad, page 244
Wholemeal wrap
Lettuce, tomatoes, bean sprouts (see box opposite), red onion

SNACK
Plums

DINNER
225g roast lean top rump

Bean, Corn and Quinoa Salad, page 248
Salad of lettuce, grated carrots, radishes and fat-free dressing

DESSERT
Apple Cinnamon Brown Rice Pudding, page 271

SNACK
Clementines

HERE'S THE LOWDOWN

Choose the bean sprouts you like best. Bean sprouts are germinated seeds that are rich in vitamins and minerals, amino acids, protein and dietary fibre. Mung beans and alfalfa sprouts are the most widely recognised types, but there are many other varieties, all with varying amounts of protein and nutritional values. Here are some of the nutritional benefits of the most common types of sprouts:

- Alfalfa sprouts: 35 per cent protein, more chlorophyll than spinach or kale, as much carotene as carrots.
- Lentil sprouts: 25 per cent protein, high in folate, great source of vitamin C and B vitamins.
- Mung bean sprouts: 20 per cent protein, great source of vitamin C, B vitamins and vitamin K.

Week 2, Day 3

6-Day Fuel Up

BREAKFAST
Apple wedges
Cucumber and yogurt dip
Smoked Salmon and Egg Open Sandwich, page 205
Coffee or tea with skimmed milk and Truvia or Splenda

SNACK
1 small handful of Craisins

LUNCH
Cashew Chicken Salad with Coriander Dressing, page 219
4 wholewheat or rye crackers

SNACK
Cantaloupe melon cubes

DINNER
225g baked chicken breast
Carrot Soup with North African Spices, page 211
Fennel, Apple and Rocket Salad, page 249

DESSERT
Sugar-free jelly

SNACK
Strawberries sprinkled with sugar substitute

Week 2, Day 4

6-Day Fuel Up

BREAKFAST
1 Sharon fruit or kiwi fruit
Breakfast Wrap, page 190
Coffee or tea with skimmed milk and Truvia or Splenda

SNACK
Pan-seared banana slices

LUNCH
Hot Black-Eyed Bean and Chicken Soup, page 210
Side salad of tomato pieces, cucumber chunks and red onion
   slices with fat-free Italian dressing
Asparagus spears, steamed

SNACK
Apple slices

DINNER
Spaghetti and Meat Sauce, page 214
Spinach, steamed

DESSERT
Mug of sugar-free hot cocoa
Sprinkle of cinnamon

SNACK
25g low-fat Cheddar cheese
2 wholewheat or rye crackers

Week 2, Day 5

6-Day Fuel Up

BREAKFAST
185g cooked quinoa
½ avocado, stoned, peeled and sliced
1 veggie burger or sausage
115g low-fat cottage cheese
Coffee or tea with skimmed milk and Truvia or Splenda

SNACK
Sliced banana

LUNCH
Asian Salad with Tuna, page 243

SNACK
Grapefruit segments

DINNER
225g baked chicken breast
Roasted Garlic Cauliflower Mash, page 256

DESSERT
250g fat-free yogurt
2 Granola Plum Mini-muffin Pastries, page 274

SNACK
Baby carrots with Savoury Yogurt Dip, page 264

HERE'S THE LOWDOWN

Enjoying an evening dessert that is filled with fibre, like Granola Plum Mini-muffin Pastries, ensures your GI tract will be running smoothly the next day.

TIME SAVER

Let your salad dressing double up as a dipping sauce for veggies. Make extra Sesame Miso Dressing to use throughout the week with your veggies.

Week 2, Day 6

6-Day Fuel Up

BREAKFAST
Mandarin orange slices and 50g rolled oats mixed into 250g fat-free Greek yogurt
Egg and Veggie Scramble, page 197
Coffee or tea with skimmed milk and Truvia or Splenda

SNACK
Vanilla Poached Pears, page 260

LUNCH
Puy Lentil Salad, page 225
115g grilled chicken breast

SNACK
Raspberry and blackberry mix

DINNER
225g grilled fillet steak
Courgette, pan-fried in olive oil spray
80g cooked bulgur wheat

DESSERT
50ml (1 small scoop) low-fat ice cream
1 Figgy Biscuit, page 273

SNACK
Grapes

TIME SAVER

Make double or triple the amount of bulgur wheat you
need, then divide into individual serving sizes and freeze.

Week 2, Day 7

6-Day Fuel Up

BREAKFAST
Garden Veggie Frittata, page 196
1 thin slice wholemeal toast
250g fat-free Greek yogurt
Coffee or tea with skimmed milk and Truvia or Splenda

SNACK
Tangerines

LUNCH
Pasta with Chicken and Fresh Summer Vegetables, page 215
Carrot and celery sticks

SNACK
Mango slices

DINNER
Old-fashioned Beef Stew, page 235
Salad with baby spinach, mandarin orange slices, fat-free dressing

DESSERT
1 serving Grandma's Low-fat Chocolate Pudding, page 279
1 tsp crystallised ginger pieces

SNACK
Tangerines

Week 3, Day 1

1-Day Power Up

After two full weeks, you are beginning to see just how fast you can burn fat and lose weight with this diet. By now, you may be noticing that your jeans don't fit as snugly as they used to, you have more energy, and you don't feel as hungry as you used to. And you're undoubtedly looking forward to today's 1-Day Power Up so that you can lose up to 2 pounds (900g) more overnight. Rest assured, you'll be doing it in delicious style.

BREAKFAST
Enchanted Blueberry Smoothie, page 182

Rich, thick and brimming with vibrant flavour, this smoothie is packed with the antioxidant power of blueberries.

LUNCH
Delightfully Spicy Smoothie, page 176

Spice up your day with a tangy smoothie that is sure to tantalise your taste buds and keep you cruising through the afternoon.

DINNER
Piña Colada Island Smoothie, page 181

Celebrate today's ending with a Piña Colada-style smoothie that puts you in the holiday mood thanks to sweet pineapple and creamy coconut.

Week 3, Day 2

6-Day Fuel Up

BREAKFAST
Grapes
Kippers on Rye with Baby Spinach, page 198
Coffee or tea with skimmed milk and Truvia or Splenda

SNACK
Apple slices

LUNCH
Tuna Delight, page 246
1 large carrot, steamed with 1 tsp butter

SNACK
Sliced banana

DINNER
Braised Fillet Steak in Mushroom and Red Wine Sauce, page 234
Side salad with 1 tbsp Lemon Caper Vinaigrette, page 267
95g cooked quinoa

DESSERT
Smart Brownies, page 277

SNACK
Cherries

Week 3, Day 3

6-Day Fuel Up

BREAKFAST
Sausage and Egg Scramble, page 202
115g low-fat cottage cheese
Coffee or tea with skimmed milk and Truvia or Splenda

SNACK
Plums

LUNCH
1 turkey wrap with: 115g turkey, 1 slice low-fat cheese,
   1 wholemeal wrap
Lettuce, tomato, onion, pickles, bean sprouts, mustard
Green beans, sautéed

SNACK
Canned fruit (in its own juice)

DINNER
Rosemary Pork Roast, page 239
Mixed salad leaves salad with Honey Garlic Balsamic
   Vinaigrette, page 267

DESSERT
Lemon Custard with Fresh Blueberry Sauce, page 278

SNACK
Melon balls

TIME SAVER

Cook an extra 225g of the Rosemary Pork Roast to save for Week 3, Day 5.

Week 3, Day 4

6-Day Fuel Up

BREAKFAST
Spicy Tofu Scramble, page 206
Coffee or tea with skimmed milk and Truvia or Splenda

SNACK
Strawberry slices sprinkled with sugar substitute (optional)

LUNCH
Open tuna salad sandwich with: tuna salad (85g tuna in water, 1 hardboiled egg, 1 tbsp extra-light mayonnaise, salt and pepper)
Sliced tomato, lettuce, bean sprouts, red onion
1 thin slice wholemeal bread

SNACK
Baked banana slices with just a drizzle of maple syrup

DINNER
Shepherd's Pie with Chicken, page 226

DESSERT
50ml (1 small scoop) low-fat ice cream
1 low-fat gingernut biscuit

SNACK
Apples with Creamy Peanut Dip, page 258

HERE'S THE LOWDOWN

Don't miss out on the health benefits and high-protein content of yogurt just because you have trouble digesting dairy products. If you experience gas, bloating or stomach pains after eating these foods, it may be due to an inability to process lactose, a type of sugar found in milk and dairy products. This is called lactose intolerance, but there's hope. Certain dairy products are naturally lower in lactose, including hard, aged cheeses, such as Cheddar, Gruyère and Parmesan; cottage cheese; and yogurts with live and active cultures. In addition, most supermarkets carry lactose-reduced or lactose-free dairy products, which minimise any digestive problems. You can also try probiotics to ease the symptoms of lactose intolerance. Kefir is a natural probiotic drink similar to a liquid yogurt that keeps your digestive system running smoothly. You can also take a supplement, such as Lactaid, that provides the enzyme lactase needed by your body to digest dairy.

TIME SAVER

Make Celeriac Remoulade tonight for tomorrow's lunch to allow the flavour to be enhanced.

Week 3, Day 5

6-Day Fuel Up

BREAKFAST
Diana's Magnificent Hearty Pancakes, page 194
250g fat-free yogurt (spread on pancake)
1 apple and 1 pear stewed with cinnamon, cloves and nutmeg
  (to top the yogurt layer)
Coffee or tea with skimmed milk and Truvia or Splenda

SNACK
Sliced banana, strawberries and blueberries

LUNCH
115g oven-baked chicken breast
Celeriac Rémoulade, page 251
1 small wholemeal roll

SNACK
Orange segments

DINNER
Rosemary Pork Roast, page 239
Courgettes, steamed

DESSERT
Grapes and Walnuts with Lemon Sauce, page 280

SNACK
Carrot, cucumber and celery sticks

> **TIME SAVER**
>
> Use the Rosemary Pork Roast you cooked on Week 3, Day 3.

Week 3, Day 6

6-Day Fuel Up

BREAKFAST
Sausage and Egg Scramble, page 202
250ml low-fat kefir or fat-free yogurt
Coffee or tea with skimmed milk and Truvia or Splenda

SNACK
Stewed apples with cinnamon and a sprinkle of sugar substitute

LUNCH
Lemon Roasted Salmon, page 242
Asparagus spears, grilled
80g cooked brown basmati rice mixed with chopped, fresh
   coriander

SNACK
Melon cubes

DINNER
Thai Chicken Noodle Soup, page 212
Thai Chicken Salad, page 231

DESSERT
Grilled Fruit with Balsamic Syrup, page 276

SNACK
1 small handful of dried fruit mixture

Week 3, Day 7

6-Day Fuel Up

BREAKFAST
2 poached eggs
250g fat-free yogurt
Coffee or tea with skimmed milk and Truvia or Splenda

SNACK
Sharon fruit or kiwi fruit

LUNCH
115g grilled prawns
Green beans, sautéed
75g soaked wholemeal couscous

SNACK
Raw cauliflower with Savoury Yogurt Dip, page 264

DINNER
Indian Spiced Chicken, page 228
Rice Pilaff, page 257
Spinach side salad with fat-free salad dressing

DESSERT
100ml (2 small scoops) fat-free frozen strawberry yogurt
Sliced strawberries

SNACK
Apple slices

Week 4, Day 1

1-Day Power Up

After just 21 days, you should be looking leaner, feeling stronger and bursting with more energy than ever before. Give yourself a pat on the back! Then spark overnight weight loss again with this delicious trio of smoothies.

BREAKFAST
Morning Sunshine Smoothie, page 178

The sweetness of mango and banana in this zingy treat immediately puts you in holiday mode. Is there a better way to start your day?

LUNCH
Tropical Medley Smoothie, page 183

This delightful drink is bursting with flavours from tropical islands – mango, coconut and banana – that will transport you to a beautifully sunny paradise. Sip away on this super-sized smoothie all afternoon.

DINNER
Kale Margarita Smoothie, page 179

What a perfect way to wind down the day. Enjoy a different kind of margarita that's smooth and sweet and is guaranteed to leave you feeling lively and energetic tomorrow morning.

Week 4, Day 2

6-Day Fuel Up

BREAKFAST
Spicy Egg Scramble, page 203
250g fat-free yogurt
Coffee or tea with skimmed milk and Truvia or Splenda

SNACK
Red peppers and green beans with fat-free dressing as a dip

LUNCH
Extra-healthy Spinach Salad with Turkey, page 224

SNACK
Fresh mango, strawberries and banana pieces

DINNER
Chicken and Veggie Stir-fry, page 221
80g cooked brown basmati rice

DESSERT
1 small pot of low-fat rice pudding
1 biscotti

SNACK
Tangerines

Week 4, Day 3

6-Day Fuel Up

BREAKFAST
Egg and Spinach Omelette, page 195
½ wholemeal sesame bagel, toasted or ½ slice wholemeal toast
Savoury Yogurt Dip, page 264
1 orange, sliced
Coffee or tea with skimmed milk and Truvia or Splenda

SNACK
Strawberries, blueberries, raspberries and blackberries drizzled
with balsamic vinegar and a pinch of muscovado sugar (optional)

LUNCH

Vegetable Stir-fry, page 237, with 115g chicken breast

SNACK

Cucumber slices, tomato wedges, red onion rings with Savoury
Yogurt Dip, page 264

DINNER

225g fillet steak
Spinach, stir-fried with garlic
Mushrooms, pan-fried
80g cooked bulgur wheat

DESSERT

Cherries with Ricotta and Toasted Almonds, page 270

SNACK

Mandarin oranges, drained if canned

TIME SAVER

Prepare Baked Burritos and Baked Cheesy Tomatoes
tonight for tomorrow's dinner. Cover with foil and put in
the fridge. When you're ready to bake, leave to stand at
room temperature for 30 minutes before popping it in
the oven.

Week 4, Day 4

6-Day Fuel Up

BREAKFAST
40–50g high-fibre cereal (unsweetened)
200ml skimmed milk
1 apple, sliced
125g fat-free Greek yogurt, mixed with ⅓ scoop protein powder
1 boiled egg
Coffee or tea with skimmed milk and Truvia or Splenda

SNACK
Mango and pineapple slushy (blend frozen fruit with ice and eat
 with a spoon)

LUNCH
Apple Tuna Wrap, page 240

SNACK
Fresh figs

DINNER
Baked Chicken Burritos, page 222
Baked Cheesy Tomatoes, page 255

DESSERT
1 small pot low-fat chocolate mousse
1 low-fat gingernut biscuit

SNACK
Grapefruit segments

Week 4, Day 5

6-Day Fuel Up

BREAKFAST
Oat 'Pudding' with Chocolate and Lime, page 201
2 eggs, scrambled
Coffee or tea with skimmed milk and Truvia or Splenda

SNACK
Baby carrots

LUNCH
Spiced Cauliflower Cheese, page 254
115g grilled chicken breast
Swiss chard, stir-fried

SNACK
Apple slices

DINNER
Miso soup
Pan-Fried Wild Salmon with Mustard Sauce, page 245
Japanese Spinach Salad, page 252

DESSERT
250ml warmed skimmed milk sprinkled with nutmeg
1 low-fat digestive biscuit

SNACK
1 peach

Week 4, Day 6

6-Day Fuel Up

BREAKFAST
2-egg veggie omelette (with spinach, mushrooms, tomatoes and
  onions)
1 thin slice wholemeal toast
2 tbsp peanut butter, no added sugar
Coffee or tea with skimmed milk and Truvia or Splenda

SNACK
Cherries
200ml low-fat hot chocolate or chocolate drink

LUNCH
Chicken, Spinach and Basil Pizza, page 218
Large Caesar salad with fat-free dressing and no croutons

SNACK
Grapes

DINNER
225g grilled fillet steak
Cauliflower, roasted
Asparagus spears, roasted

DESSERT
100ml (2 small scoops) fat-free frozen yogurt
1 tbsp fat-free chocolate syrup (see page 138)

SNACK
Fresh veggie sticks and Savoury Yogurt Dip, page 264

Week 4, Day 7

6-DAY FUEL UP

BREAKFAST
30g rolled oats, cooked
1 tbsp raisins
Egg and Veggie Scramble, page 197
Coffee or tea with skimmed milk and Truvia or Splenda

SNACK
Sliced banana with a sprinkle of cinnamon, toasted lightly

LUNCH
Tomato and basil soup, canned or from a carton
1 wholemeal pitta stuffed with:
Spicy Meatballs, page 232
Mixed leaf salad with tomatoes
Condiments: mustard, horseradish, pickles, capers

SNACK
Cucumbers, tomatoes and celery with fat-free Italian dressing
for dipping

DINNER
Berry, Carrot and Apple Salad, page 247
225g roast turkey breast

DESSERT
1 chocolate brownie, 5cm square
100ml (2 small scoops) fat-free frozen yogurt

SNACK
Strawberries

CHAPTER SEVEN

....

1-Day Power Up Recipes

The jumbo smoothie recipes here will keep you feeling refreshed, energised and satisfied as you burn fat and boost your overall health. Lead nutritionist at the Nutrition and Weight Management Center at Boston Medical Center, Diana Cullum-Dugan, took on the challenge to help come up with 25 smoothie recipes to include in this book, and it was a tall order. To maximise the 1-Day Power Up's potential to jump-start weight loss, each smoothie had to meet some very exacting specifications, including:

- Providing protein to maintain lean muscle
- Rich fibre content to promote smooth digestion and to keep you feeling pleasantly full for hours
- Using wholesome, good-for-your-health foods
- Using everyday ingredients you can easily find
- Taking less than 3 minutes to make
- And, most importantly, being undeniably, unequivocally, lip-smackingly delicious

The smoothies you'll find here succeeded beyond all expectations on every count. Of course, all of the smoothies underwent rigorous taste testing. Smoothie taste-testing day turned out to be a real favourite at the Center. Week after week, doctors, nurses and support staff members would all crowd around to get a taste of the samples. The funny thing is that everybody had very different preferences. Some people fell in love with the refreshing fruity varieties like Enchanted Blueberry and Crispy Apple. One of the nurses always went back for seconds of the savoury flavours, like Delightfully Spicy, which has a little kick to it. And one of the assistants couldn't stop raving about the thick, creamy dessert-like smoothies with hints of chocolate (Spa Crazy Chocolate) or peanut butter (Peanut Butter Cup).

You'll find something you love too. Whether you gravitate towards spicy, savoury or sweet, you'll discover sinlessly delicious recipes to suit your taste. Some patients like a fruity creation in the morning, something a little more savoury for lunch and a sweet treat in the evening. You are encouraged to aim for variety by choosing three different smoothies throughout the day, rather than sticking with the same one morning, noon and night. To make it easy, we've created the selection chart on page 175, with instructions on choosing your smoothies if you want to stray from the plan outlined in Chapter 6. You can experiment with new smoothies each week or stick with your favourites. Try a few, or try them all. It's up to you.

How to choose your smoothies

For your first four 1-Day Power Up days, you must choose one smoothie from Column 1, one smoothie from Column 2, and one Smoothie from Column 3 of the Smoothie Selection Chart rather than having three smoothies from a single column on a single day. You can have your three smoothies in any order you like throughout the course of your 1-Day Power Up; just be sure to pick one from each of the first three columns. *Note:* Because the Physicians Protein Smoothie provides an ideal blend of nutrients, it's OK to have it three times a day if you wish – stick to your favourite flavour or mix them up. (For this reason, it is listed in each column.)

If you want to make your own smoothie, you may replace one smoothie from Column 3 with one of your own creation using the Mix 'n' Match Smoothie Chart in Appendix A.

After the first four weeks on the Overnight Diet, you have more options:

- Continue to choose one smoothie from each of the first three columns.

- Continue to choose one smoothie from Columns 1 and 2 and create one of your own in place of one in Column 3.

- Swap one smoothie from Column 3 for a smoothie in Column 4.

- If you would prefer having only two smoothies a day instead of three, you can choose one from Column 3 and one from Column 4.

All of these smoothies are big in size, flavour and fat-burning power. What makes them even better is that you can whip them up in mere moments. Grab a handful of ingredients, toss them in a blender and press a button. What could be easier? If you're a busy parent or you are constantly on the go, you need something that's lightning-fast to prepare. You won't find anything that's quicker or easier to make that will give you the overnight results you want. They're economical too, so they won't lighten your wallet much while they're lightening your weight.

The recipes that follow list ingredients, followed by simple instructions. If you wish to see how easy it is to make them, you can find a video demonstration at OvernightDiet.co.uk. If you

Smoothie Selection Chart

Column 1	Column 2	Column 3	Column 4
Banana Latte	Kale Margarita	Crispy Apple	Blueberry Freeze
Delightfully Spicy	Orange Zest	Enchanted Blueberry	California Dreaming
Green Machine	Chocolate Banana Swirl	Green Apple Goddess	Cherry Jubilee
Morning Sunshine	Piña Colada Island	Tropical Medley	Figtastic
Physicians Protein Smoothie	Physicians Protein Smoothie	Physicians Protein Smoothie	Key Lime Pie
		(or your own creation using the 'Mix 'n' Match Smoothie Chart')	Mango Madness
			Mint Melody
			Peanut Butter Cup
			Punchy Pomegranate
			Really Clean and Green
			Spa Crazy Chocolate
			Spicy First Date
			Strawberry Fields
			Physicians Protein Smoothie

want even more recipes, visit the website or Facebook page (www.facebook/dr.caroline.apovian), where you'll find additional recipes from patients and from other readers. Feel free to join the conversation and share your own recipes there too.

Important! You do not have to adjust the protein amounts in the smoothie recipes to your DPR. The DPR is strictly for the 6-Day Fuel Up.

Banana Latte

....

Everybody loves a latte. This banana-flavoured coffee smoothie is so good, and you definitely can't get it at your local coffee shop. Enjoy it as a healthy pick-me-up any time of day.

Protein: 1 scoop protein powder (see pages 64–5)
250ml skimmed milk
175ml strong black coffee (decaf is fine)
2 bananas, sliced
a handful of ice cubes

Put all the ingredients into a blender or food processor and blend until smooth.

Delightfully Spicy

....

Filled with spicy and silky notes (rocket peppers the palate and avocado is creamy and smooth), this tangy smoothie is sure to spice up your day. Add crushed chilli flakes for a more intense bite.

Protein: 1 scoop protein powder (see pages 64–5)

1 large pepper (red, orange or yellow)

2 oranges, peeled and quartered

1 celery stick

1 small, ripe avocado, stoned, peeled and sliced

20g rocket

350ml water

¼ tsp crushed chilli flakes (optional)

Put all the ingredients into a blender or food processor and blend until smooth.

HELP!

My smoothie's too thick

If your smoothie comes out thicker than you would like, simply add a little water to give it a thinner consistency. In general, if you prefer a smoothie that's closer to a juice in consistency, use fresh produce rather than frozen, and use water rather than ice.

My smoothie's too watery

If you've made your smoothie and it comes out thinner than you would like, just add small amounts of ice until it reaches the thickness you desire. If you tend to prefer a thicker smoothie, try using frozen fruits and veggies. That really helps create a thick and creamy consistency.

Remember, for any of these recipes, you can use fresh or frozen fruits and veggies.

Green Machine

....

Going green has never been more delicious! Add the tomato and the celery, and you just might think you're enjoying a virgin Bloody Mary.

Protein: 250g fat-free Greek yogurt
1 handful of ice cubes
½ cucumber, peeled and sliced
1 carrot, sliced
1 small tomato, quartered
1 celery stick, sliced
2 handfuls of spinach
salt and freshly ground black pepper

Put all the ingredients into a blender or food processor and blend until smooth.

Morning Sunshine

....

Nothing says 'good morning' like sunshine. Sweetness pulsates from prunes, mango and banana. You can have your morning sunshine any time of day – for breakfast, lunch or dinner.

Protein: 1 scoop protein powder (see pages 64–5)
5 stoned prunes
½ banana, sliced
165g mango, peeled and diced
2 handfuls of spinach

Put all the ingredients into a blender or food processor and blend until smooth.

Kale Margarita

....

There's nothing like a margarita to make your day. Bitter kale, sweet mango and succulent coconut water make up for the lack of tequila.

  Protein: 1 scoop protein powder (see pages 64–5)
  2–3 handfuls chopped and stemmed kale
  325g mango, peeled, stoned and cubed
  360ml prepared margarita mix (such as Jose Cuervo brand)
  120–175ml coconut water, as needed
  1 handful of ice cubes

Put all the ingredients into a blender or food processor and blend until smooth.

Orange Zest

....

Juice up your day with this ever-popular citrus fruit.

  Protein: 1 scoop protein powder (see pages 64–5)
  zest of 1 orange
  1 seedless orange, quartered (including the flesh and pith)
  ½ banana, sliced
  1 plum, stoned
  juice of 1 whole lemon
  3 large Swiss chard leaves, stemmed

Put all the ingredients into a blender or food processor and blend until smooth.

Chocolate Banana Swirl

························

Banana, chocolate and cinnamon make a satisfying and spicy creation.

Protein: 1 scoop protein powder (see pages 64–5)
1 banana, sliced
1 tbsp fat-free chocolate syrup (see page 138)
½ tsp cinnamon
250ml skimmed milk
1 handful of ice cubes

Put all the ingredients into a blender or food processor and blend until smooth.

MILKS

In recipes that call for milk, both here and in Chapter 8, you should stick to skimmed or semi-skimmed if you're using cow's milk. Always feel free to substitute with unsweetened almond milk or soya milk if you prefer.

Piña Colada Island

....

When you want something sweet, try this smoothie filled with chunks of pineapple, creamy coconut and naturally wholesome agave nectar.

Protein: 250g fat-free Greek yogurt
165g pineapple chunks (fresh or canned in water or its own juice)
1 banana, sliced
½ tsp vanilla extract
1 tsp agave nectar
about 1 handful of ice cubes (add more as needed for consistency)

Put all the ingredients into a blender or food processor and blend until smooth.

Crispy Apple

....

Give this juicy smoothie a twist by going for a tart Granny Smith apple, or make a sweeter version with a red apple.

Protein: 1 scoop protein powder (see pages 64–5)
250ml water
1 apple, cored and quartered
1 orange, peeled and quartered
1 banana, sliced
2 handfuls of spinach
1 carrot, sliced

Put all the ingredients into a blender or food processor and blend until smooth.

Enchanted Blueberry

....

You'll be enchanted by this blueberry-infused treat that sneaks in some good-for-you veggies.

Protein: 1 scoop protein powder (see pages 64–5)
185g fat-free blueberry yogurt
1 banana, sliced
2 handfuls of spinach
150g blueberries
2 handfuls of ice cubes

Put all the ingredients into a blender or food processor and blend until smooth.

Green Apple Goddess

....

This smoothie is almost like having a whole fruit basket in a blender.

Protein: 1 scoop protein powder (see pages 64–5)
1 green apple, cored and quartered
75g blueberries
165g pineapple, diced (fresh or canned in water or its own juice)
125g raspberries
1–2 handfuls of spinach
½ cos or Romaine lettuce
2 large kale leaves, stemmed and chopped
2 stoned dried dates
475ml water

Put all the ingredients into a blender or food processor and blend until smooth.

Tropical Medley

....

Prepare your taste buds for a mouth-watering mix of island-inspired flavours.

Protein: 1 scoop protein powder (see pages 64–5)
1 banana, sliced
85g mango, peeled and diced
50ml light, unsweetened coconut milk
250ml water
3 handfuls of Swiss chard or baby spinach (stemmed if
   necessary)
1 tsp vanilla extract

Put all the ingredients into a blender or food processor and blend until smooth.

Blueberry Freeze

....

Frozen blueberries and banana add creamy thickness to this fruity delight, while agave nectar lends wholesome, natural sweetness.

Protein: 250g fat-free Greek yogurt
1 banana, sliced
120ml skimmed milk
1½ tsp ground flaxseed
1 tsp agave nectar
150g frozen blueberries

Put all the ingredients into a blender or food processor and blend until smooth.

California Dreaming

....

If you're dreaming about being ready for bikini season, this peachy smoothie will help to make that dream a reality.

Protein: 250g fat-free Greek yogurt
1 peach
145g strawberries
1 banana, sliced
2 tbsp ground flaxseed
3 handfuls of ice cubes

Put all the ingredients into a blender or food processor and blend until smooth.

Cherry Jubilee

....

Delectable ripe cherries in season make this a celebration-worthy smoothie.

Protein: 1 scoop protein powder (see pages 64–5)
1–2 bananas, sliced
150g cherries, stoned
475ml water
1 handful of spinach

Put all the ingredients into a blender or food processor and blend until smooth.

Figtastic

....

Fantastic fibre-rich figs provide the foundation for this one-of-a-kind creation, while hints of cinnamon and vanilla give it even more flair.

Protein: 1 scoop protein powder (see pages 64–5)
4–5 fresh figs
150g red seedless grapes
250ml water
1 handful of ice cubes
½ tsp ground cinnamon
½ tsp vanilla extract

Put all the ingredients into a blender or food processor and blend until smooth.

Key Lime Pie

....

If you've ever tasted a Key Lime Pie, you'll love the refreshing good-ness of this smoothie. Zesty lime combines with tropical coconut for a taste explosion.

Protein: 1 scoop protein powder (see pages 64–5)
zest and juice of 1 lime
250ml light, unsweetened coconut milk
1 tbsp coconut oil
1 banana, sliced
1 tsp agave nectar
2 tbsp rolled oats
1 tsp vanilla extract

Put all the ingredients into a blender or food processor and blend until smooth.

Mango Madness

....

Bursting with the juicy sweetness of mango, this smoothie also holds a hint of savoury in the form of rocket and spinach.

Protein: 1 scoop protein powder (see pages 64–5)
1 banana, sliced
1 orange, peeled and quartered
1 handful of rocket
2 handfuls of spinach
1 peach
325g mango, peeled and cubed
2 stoned dried dates
250–475ml water, as needed

Put all the ingredients into a blender or food processor and blend until smooth.

Mint Melody

....

Refreshingly cool and highly flavourful, this minty smoothie perks you up and puts a little pep in your step.

Protein: 1 scoop protein powder (see pages 64–5)
330g pineapple, cubed (fresh or canned in water or its own juice)
2 bananas, sliced
1 handful of mint leaves
250ml water

Put all the ingredients into a blender or food processor and blend until smooth.

Peanut Butter Cup

....

Ever had a Peanut Butter Cup in a glass? That's what this amazing dessert-like smoothie tastes like.

Protein: 250g fat-free Greek yogurt
120ml skimmed milk
1 tbsp fat-free chocolate syrup (see page 138)
1 tbsp reduced-fat smooth peanut butter, no added sugar
1 banana, sliced

Put all the ingredients into a blender or food processor and blend until smooth.

Punchy Pomegranate

....

Pomegranates have been heralded for generations for their divine flavour and health benefits.

Protein: 1 scoop protein powder (see pages 64–5)
120ml pomegranate juice
1 handful of kale, Swiss chard or spinach, stemmed if
   necessary
1 banana, sliced
40g strawberries
75g blueberries
1 tbsp ground flaxseed
50ml skimmed milk

Put all the ingredients into a blender or food processor and blend until smooth.

Really Green and Clean

....

Enjoy a delightful blend of sweet freshness and savoury goodness that will leave you feeling energized and ready to go.

Protein: 1 scoop protein powder (see pages 64–5)
2 carrots, sliced
1 apple, cored and quartered
2 soft or semi-dried dates, stoned
1 banana, sliced
85g mango, peeled and diced
2 handfuls of spinach or kale (stemmed if necessary)
about 250ml water (add more as needed)

Put all the ingredients into a blender or food processor and blend until smooth.

Spa Crazy Chocolate

....

You'll go crazy for this chocolate–coconut combo – you might think it came from the local ice cream shop!

Protein: 1 scoop protein powder (see pages 64–5)
120ml unsweetened coconut milk
½ tsp blackstrap molasses
2 tbsp Truvia or Splenda
2 tbsp unsweetened cocoa powder
1 banana, sliced
½ ripe avocado, stoned, peeled and sliced
1 small carrot, sliced
1 small celery stick, sliced
1 handful of spinach
2 handfuls of ice cubes

Put all the ingredients into a blender or food processor and blend until smooth.

Spicy First Date

....

In the mood for a hint of spice? Savour sweetly delicious, decidedly exotic dates enveloped in the intoxicating scent of vanilla along with overtones of ginger, cloves and chilli.

Protein: 250g fat-free Greek yogurt

4 stoned dried dates

1 banana, sliced

250ml skimmed milk

½ tsp vanilla extract

½–1 tsp cinnamon, to taste

a pinch each of ground ginger, ground cloves, freshly grated nutmeg, chilli powder and chilli pepper

1 handful of ice cubes

Put all the ingredients into a blender or food processor and blend until smooth.

Strawberry Fields

....

Take just one sip of this smoothie and you'll understand why strawberries are the most popular berry in the world.

Protein: 1 scoop protein powder (see pages 64–5)

75g strawberries

125g fat-free vanilla yogurt

50ml fresh orange juice

Put all the ingredients into a blender or food processor and blend until smooth.

CHAPTER EIGHT

....

6-Day Fuel Up Recipes

BREAKFASTS

Breakfast Wrap

....

Preparation time: **5 minutes** | Cooking time: **2 minutes**
Serves **1** | Protein per serving towards DPR: **60g**

This tasty, simple breakfast provides a protein boost that keeps you feeling full all morning long.

Protein: 2 eggs, adjust to your DPR
30cm wholemeal wrap
½ bunch watercress, leaves only
balsamic vinegar
small pack of asparagus tips, chopped in half
salt and freshly ground pepper to taste

1. Place the wrap on a plate, place the watercress leaves on one side of the wrap and sprinkle with a little balsamic vinegar.

2. Spray a small non-stick pan with olive oil, place over a medium heat, add the eggs and scramble until cooked through. Meanwhile, blanch the asparagus tips in boiling water then drain.

3. Place the scrambled eggs and the asparagus tips over the watercress, season to taste and roll your wrap.

Poached Eggs and Beans

....

Preparation time: **5 minutes** | Cooking time: **5 minutes**
Serves **1** | Protein per serving towards DPR: **60g**

Protein combined with fibre from the beans and whole grains increase satiety to stave off hunger

Protein: 2 eggs, adjust to your DPR
150g can sugar-free baked beans
oil spray
1 thin slice wholemeal soda bread
handful of mushrooms, chopped

1. Poach the eggs in the microwave, following the manufacturer's instructions, or use a poacher on the hob. Heat the beans in a small pan over a gentle heat.

2. Spray a small frying pan with the oil and fry the mushrooms until cooked, about 5 minutes.

3. Toast the soda bread then serve topped with the eggs and accompanied by the beans and mushrooms.

WHOLE EGGS AND EGG WHITES – CONTRIBUTION TO DPR

Remember, whole eggs and egg whites make a valuable contribution to your DPR, particularly at breakfast. One large egg contributes approximately 30g towards your total daily amount of protein; the whites of 2 large eggs contribute the same amount.

Crustless Quiche

Preparation time: **10–15 minutes** | Cooking time: **30 minutes**
Serves **4** | Protein per serving towards DPR: **60g**

Who needs crust? The rich creaminess of eggs and feta cheese mixed with spinach makes this a favourite! Note that if you make this on Monday, you could have three pieces left over to grab and go throughout the week.

Protein: 3 large eggs plus whites of 2 eggs, adjust to your DPR
Protein: 115g sliced ham, diced, adjust to your DPR
oil spray
1 tsp olive oil
1 onion, finely chopped
175g baby spinach
75g plain wholemeal flour
½ tsp baking powder
¼ tsp salt
320ml skimmed milk
⅛ tsp cayenne pepper
salt and freshly ground black pepper
75g low-fat feta cheese

1. Preheat the oven to 200°C/400°F/Gas 6. Spray a 25cm pie dish with oil spray. Heat the olive oil in a medium frying pan over medium heat and cook the onion for 5 minutes or until soft, stirring frequently. Add the spinach and cook for 1–2 minutes until wilted. Set aside.

2. In a large bowl, whisk together the eggs, egg whites, flour, baking powder and salt. Whisk in the milk until just blended. Stir in the spinach and onion mixture and the ham. Season with the cayenne pepper and salt and pepper.

3. Pour the mixture into the pie dish, top with the feta cheese and bake for 25 minutes or until the centre is set and the edge is golden brown. Leave to set for 5 minutes before slicing and serving.

Peanut Butter and Raisin Wrap

Preparation time: **5 minutes** | Makes: **1 serving**

Variations on this simple, hearty combination are a great favourite with kids of all ages in the States. It might sound unusual, but give it go – you'll be pleasantly surprised.

30cm wholemeal wrap
2 tbsp natural, no-sugar peanut butter
2 tbsp raisins
½ banana, sliced

Spread the wrap with the peanut butter, top with raisins and banana slices and roll it up.

Diana's Magnificent Hearty Pancakes

....

Preparation time: **10 minutes** | Cooking time: **20 minutes**
Makes: **12** (Serving size: **2** pancakes) | Protein per serving
towards DPR: **60g**

Who says you can't eat pancakes and lose weight? Eggs, protein powder and whole grains turn these pancakes into a powerfully delicious weight-loss ally. Serve them right out of the pan!

> Protein: 240g protein powder (see pages 64–5), adjust to
>   your DPR
> Protein: 4 eggs plus whites of 2 eggs, adjust to your DPR
> 300g plain wholemeal flour
> 1 tbsp ground flaxseed
> 50g rolled oats
> 60g plain white flour
> 2 tbsp baking powder
> 540ml skimmed milk
> 2 tbsp olive oil
> oil spray

1. Mix together all dry ingredients in a large bowl. Mix together the eggs, egg whites, milk and oil in a separate bowl.

2. Pour the egg mixture into the dry ingredients, then use a spatula or spoon to stir from the base of the bowl until all the dry ingredients are moistened. Do not over-mix.

3. Put a griddle or 30cm frying pan over medium heat. Spray lightly with oil spray. Pour 125ml batter into the hot pan. Cook the pancake for 3–4 minutes on the first side, or until the edge begins to dry and bubbles appear in the centre of the pancake, then flip the pancake over. Cook until lightly golden, then

remove from the pan and keep warm. Cook the remaining batter in the same way. The remaining pancakes may not take quite as long to cook, as the pan begins to maintain heat.

Egg and Spinach Omelette

....

Preparation time: **5 minutes** | Cooking time: **5 minutes**
Serves **1** | Protein per serving towards DPR: **60g**

Experiment by varying the amount of spinach (the more the better), or get creative and toss in other vegetables, too.

> Protein: 2 eggs, adjust to your DPR
> oil spray
> 25g low-fat mozzarella cheese, grated
> about 1 handful of baby spinach
> fat-free salsa, unlimited
> 1 tbsp low-fat crème fraîche (optional)

1. In a small bowl, beat the eggs until fluffy. Spray a small non-stick frying pan with oil spray and heat over medium heat.

2. Add the eggs to the pan and allow to cook until halfway set. Use the edge of a spatula to lift the edge of the omelette from the side of the pan and tilt the pan to let the uncooked egg run underneath the omelette. Continue lifting and tilting until the egg is nearly cooked through.

3. Add the grated cheese to one side of the omelette and top with the spinach. Using the spatula, lift one side of the omelette and fold it over the cheese and spinach. Cook for another 1–2 minutes until the cheese has melted. Top with liberal amounts of salsa and low-fat crème fraîche, if you like.

Garden Veggie Frittata

....

Preparation time: **20 minutes** | Cooking time: **35 minutes**
Serves **6** | Protein per serving towards DPR: **60g**

Elegant enough for brunch with friends, yet simple enough for a weekday morning meal, this frittata gives you time to get ready for your day while it cooks.

Protein: 12 large eggs, adjust to your DPR
450g asparagus, woody ends removed
1 tbsp olive oil
175g chestnut mushrooms, sliced
1 garlic clove, crushed
1 shallot, finely chopped
75ml skimmed milk
1 tsp salt
¼ tsp freshly ground black pepper
a pinch of freshly grated nutmeg
1 tbsp chopped fresh chives
1 small courgette, halved lengthways and sliced thinly
oil spray
1 large tomato, seeded and thinly sliced
2 tbsp freshly grated Parmesan cheese

1. Preheat the oven to 180°C/350°F/Gas 4. Cut the asparagus spears diagonally into 2.5cm pieces. Put into boiling water for 1–2 minutes, then immediately plunge into cold water to halt the cooking. Drain and set aside.

2. Heat the olive oil in a frying pan and fry the mushrooms over medium heat for 5–8 minutes until they soften. Add the garlic and shallot to the mushrooms and continue to cook for 3–4 minutes more. Remove the mushroom mixture from the heat and set aside.

3. In a large bowl, beat together the eggs, milk, salt, pepper, nutmeg and chives. Add the asparagus, mushroom mixture and courgette.

4. Lightly spray a 2-litre baking dish with oil spray. Pour the egg and vegetable mixture into the dish, then arrange the tomato on top. Sprinkle Parmesan cheese over and bake for 30–35 minutes until set.

Egg and Veggie Scramble

Preparation time: **5 minutes** | Cooking time: **5 minutes**
Serves **1** | Protein per serving towards DPR: **60g**

Fresh eggs, baby spinach and tomatoes ripe off the vine equals yummy protein-packed power! Add more vegetables any time you like.

Protein: 2 eggs, adjust to your DPR
oil spray
1 handful (or more) of baby spinach
1 small tomato, diced
fat-free salsa, unlimited (optional)

1. Heat a small frying pan coated with oil spray over medium heat and scramble the eggs until nearly cooked through.

2. Add the baby spinach to the pan and continue to cook until the eggs are completely done and the spinach is wilted. Serve the eggs topped with chopped tomato and with spoonfuls of salsa alongside, if you like.

Kippers on Rye with Baby Spinach

....

Preparation time: **2 minutes** | Cooking time: **3–4 minutes**
Serves **1** | Protein per serving towards DPR: **60g**

This is a lovely, satisfying treat for breakfast – and so easy to prepare too.

Protein: 60g undyed kipper fillet, adjust to your DPR
1 large tomato, halved
small bag baby spinach
1 thin slice rye bread

1. Heat the grill to medium and grill the kippers and tomato until the kipper is heated thorough without burning its delicate oils.

2. Steam the baby spinach and toast the rye bread. Place the spinach on the rye toast, top with the kipper and serve with the tomatoes.

Overnight Power Oats

....

Preparation time: **8–9 hours** | Cooking time: **5 minutes**
Serves **4** | Protein per serving towards DPR: about **60g**,
but depends on brand – check nutrition label

Love porridge but just don't have time to cook it? You can use rolled oats and soak them overnight, then just heat them through in the morning. If you have a slow cooker, this high-fibre porridge cooks overnight while you sleep. The addition of protein powder makes the porridge even more satisfying.

Protein: ¾ scoop protein powder (see page 64–5), adjust to
  your DPR
30g rolled oats
2 tbsp dried cranberries, raisins and/or chopped apricots
skimmed milk, as needed to thin
1 piece of fresh fruit of your choice (sliced banana, diced apple
  or peach)
a pinch each of ground cinnamon, ground cloves, freshly
  grated nutmeg, ground ginger, or to taste

1. Combine the oats with 1 of litre water in a medium bowl.
   Cover and chill overnight. The next morning transfer to a
   pan and heat over low heat until softened. Add the dried fruit
   and protein powder and stir in enough milk to your preferred
   consistency. Serve with the fresh fruit, sprinkled with spices.

2. Alternatively, use a slow cooker and use pinhead oatmeal
   instead of rolled oats. Combine all the ingredients in a 2-litre
   slow cooker with 1 litre water. Before bed, cover and set to
   cook on low heat for 8–9 hours. The following morning, stir
   and divide into 4 portions.

OTHER PROTEIN SOURCES

Eggs and salmon are both healthy sources of protein for
breakfast but why not try a few alternatives? Prawns are
a real treat – they're meaty yet subtle in flavour so are a
great way to follow up cereal in order to meet your DPR
for breakfast. Ham, particularly mild hams such as Serrano,
is also a good choice to follow cereal or go with eggs.
And don't forget cooked chicken and turkey, which are
convenient follow-ups for cereal and fruit breakfasts, to help
meet your DPR.

Fruit Yogurt Parfait

....

Preparation time: **5 minutes** | Serves **1**

Enjoy decadent layers of thick yogurt, fruit and honey with raw oats, making it a healthy muesli breakfast. Although the yogurt adds some protein it doesn't count towards your DPR so remember to adjust for this at your other meals.

fresh mixed fruit
375g fat-free Greek yogurt
a drizzle of honey
50g rolled oats

Put a layer of fruit in the base of a tall glass, then spoon in some yogurt, a drizzle of honey and a layer of the oats. Alternate with layers of fruit, yogurt, honey and oats, ending with oats.

Oat 'Pudding' with Chocolate and Lime

....

Preparation time: **10–15 minutes** | Cooking time: **20 minutes**
Serves **4**

Having a pudding doesn't mean it will add to your waistline. This high-fibre dessert has a punch of lime and a sweet hint of chocolate and is a real treat at breakfast if you have a sweet tooth. Follow this dish with a couple of scrambled eggs for a protein boost.

300ml skimmed milk
175ml canned light coconut milk
75g quick-cooking pinhead oatmeal
2 tbsp muscovado sugar
2 tbsp lime juice
25g dark chocolate (at least 70 per cent cocoa solids), grated
¾ tsp finely grated lime zest

1. In a medium pan, combine the milk, coconut milk and oatmeal. Bring to a simmer over medium-high heat and stir occasionally to prevent burning. Reduce the heat to low and simmer, stirring constantly, for 5–8 minutes to make a thin mixture.

2. Remove from the heat and stir in the sugar and lime juice. Leave to stand in the pan, uncovered, for 10 minutes or until slightly thickened.

3. Transfer to dessert bowls and top with the grated chocolate and lime zest. Serve warm, or at room temperature or chilled.

Sausage and Egg Scramble

....

Preparation time: **5 minutes** | Cooking time: **10 minutes**
Serves **4** | Protein per serving towards DPR: **60g**

The all-time favourite – sausage and eggs – has a mini-makeover.

Protein: 3 large eggs plus whites of 2 eggs, adjust to your DPR
Protein: 115g extra lean pork sausage, adjust to your DPR
3 tbsp skimmed milk
55g low-fat Cheddar cheese, grated

1. Remove the casing from the sausage. Put the sausage in a medium non-stick frying pan over medium heat and cook, breaking it up with a spoon, until nearly cooked through.

2. In a bowl, whisk together the eggs, egg whites and milk, then add to the sausage in the pan. Stir until the eggs and sausage are cooked through, and then top with the cheese. Leave to set for 1–2 minutes to melt the cheese.

Spicy Egg Scramble

....

Preparation time: **5 minutes** | Cooking time: **10 minutes**
Serves **4** | Protein per serving towards DPR: **60g**

Begin your day with this protein powerhouse. Spicing it up helps to boost your metabolism.

Protein: 8 eggs, adjust to your DPR
3 tbsp butter
3 large garlic cloves, crushed
2.5cm piece fresh root ginger, peeled and grated
1 bunch of spring onions, chopped
1 chilli, seeded and finely chopped (use less if you prefer
    less heat)
salt and freshly ground black pepper
5 tbsp chopped fresh coriander
crushed chilli flakes or Tabasco sauce to taste (if you want
    more heat)

1. Heat the butter in a non-stick medium frying pan over medium-high heat. Add the garlic, ginger, spring onions, chilli and a pinch of salt and pepper. Cook, stirring occasionally, for 3 minutes or until the garlic begins to brown and the mixture is fragrant. Remove from the heat and leave to cool.

2. Beat the eggs in a medium bowl, then return the pan to medium-high heat and pour in the eggs. Stir occasionally, until the eggs are almost cooked through, then remove from the heat. Stir in the fresh coriander and serve warm.

Spicy Tofu and Spinach Wrap

....

Preparation time: **5 minutes** | Cooking time: **10 minutes**
Serves **4** | Protein per serving towards DPR: **30g**

A tofu wrap is quick and easy, plus it provides protein and is rich in calcium.

> Protein: 340g tofu, drained and cut into 2.5cm cubes, adjust
>   to your DPR
> 3 tbsp extra virgin olive oil
> ½ onion, chopped
> 3 garlic cloves, crushed
> 1 tsp soy sauce
> ½ red pepper, seeded and diced
> 75g chestnut mushrooms, sliced
> 2 spring onions, sliced
> 2 tomatoes, seeded and finely chopped
> ½ tsp ground ginger
> ½ tsp chilli powder
> ¼ tsp crushed chilli flakes
> 175g baby spinach
> 4 wholemeal tortillas or chapattis
> salt and freshly ground black pepper

1. Heat the olive oil in a heavy frying pan over medium-high heat. Add the onion and garlic, and fry for 4–5 minutes until the onions begin to soften.

2. Add the soy sauce, tofu, pepper, mushrooms, spring onions, tomatoes, ginger, chilli powder and chilli flakes. Stir frequently and fry for 8–10 minutes until the vegetables are cooked and the tofu is lightly fried. Add the spinach and stir-fry for 1–2 minutes until wilted. Season with salt and pepper.

3. Divide the mixture into four servings and spoon onto the wholemeal tortillas. Roll up or fold to eat.

Smoked Salmon and Egg Open Sandwich

....

Preparation time: **5 minutes** | Cooking time: **5 minutes**
Serves **1** | Protein per serving towards DPR: **60g**

Quick and easy, yet elegant and tasty.

Protein: 25g smoked salmon, adjust to your DPR
Protein: 1 egg, adjust to your DPR
oil spray
½ small bagel
2 tsp light soft cheese

1. Heat a small frying pan sprayed with oil spray over medium heat and scramble the egg. While scrambling the egg, toast the bagel half and spread with soft cheese.

2. Layer the bagel with the scrambled egg and top with the smoked salmon.

Spicy Tofu Scramble

....

Preparation time: **10 minutes** | Cooking time: **15 minutes**
Serves **4** | Protein per serving towards DPR: **60g**

Piquant is not a word most people would give tofu, but this breakfast cannot be described in any other way.

Protein: 680g firm tofu, drained and rinsed, adjust to
your DPR
2 tbsp extra virgin olive oil
2 onions, chopped
1 garlic clove, crushed
½ red pepper, seeded and diced
35g mushrooms, sliced
1½ tbsp Dijon mustard
2 tbsp white miso
½ tbsp dried tarragon
2 tsp curry powder
½ tsp chilli powder
30g soya cheese, grated (optional)
salt and freshly ground black pepper

1. Heat the oil in a large frying pan over medium-high heat. Add the onions and fry for 3–5 minutes until soft. Add the garlic, pepper and mushrooms and fry for a further 5 minutes.

2. Meanwhile, crumble the tofu, then add it to the vegetable mixture. In a small bowl, whisk together the mustard, miso and 2 tbsp water, then pour over the mixture. Stir in the herbs and spices, then heat through for 5 minutes. Add the cheese, if using. Cover and leave the cheese to melt.

SOUPS

Hummus and Pesto Soup

....

Preparation time: **15 minutes** | Cooking time: **10 minutes**
Serves **4–6**

For a high-fibre and filling meal that's quick, this soup is made with canned chickpeas.

   3 x 400g cans chickpeas, drained and rinsed
   1.5 litres low-salt vegetable stock
   1 small chilli, seeded and diced
   3 tbsp olive oil
   juice of 2 lemons
   3 tbsp tahini
   3 small garlic cloves, crushed
   2 tsp ground cumin
   2 tsp ground coriander
   2 tsp turmeric
   salt and freshly ground black pepper
   6 tbsp basil or coriander pesto
   Garlic Pitta Chips, to serve (see page 253)

1. Put all the ingredients, except the pesto, in a large blender or food processor and blend until smooth, then transfer to a large pan. You may need to do this in batches.

2. Bring to a slow boil over medium-high heat, then simmer over low heat until heated through, stirring occasionally. Ladle the soup into shallow bowls and top with the pesto. Serve with 2–3 pitta chips per person.

Haricot Bean and Kale Soup

....

Preparation time: **10 minutes** | Cooking time: **1½ hours**
Serves **4**

Filled with antioxidants and filling fibre, kale is at its best when simmered slowly.

    1 large bunch of kale
    260g haricot beans, soaked overnight, rinsed and drained
    3 garlic cloves, peeled and left whole
    1 large shallot, peeled and left whole
    3 bay leaves
    2 litres vegetable stock
    freshly ground black pepper
    1 tbsp seasoning mix
    juice of ½ lemon
    1 tsp salt
    1 tbsp tomato purée
    1 tsp crushed chilli flakes

1. Hold each stem of kale while you pull the leaves off; discard the stems. Stack the leaves and roll them together in a bunch, then slice through into ribbons; chill until needed.

2. Put the haricot beans, garlic, shallot, bay leaves and vegetable stock into a pan and bring to the boil. Simmer for 1 hour or until almost tender. Add the pepper and seasoning mix and continue cooking for 30 minutes or until tender.

3. Put the kale in a large mixing bowl. Add the lemon juice and salt, and scrunch with your hands for 5 minutes to break down the fibres. This will reduce the kale to about half its volume. Add the kale, tomato purée and chilli flakes to the pan and simmer over low heat for 15 minutes or until tender.

Spinach Garlic Soup

....

Preparation time: **25 minutes** | Cooking time: **10 minutes**
Serves **4**

Puréed soups are an Overnight Diet favourite because they disguise the flavour of vegetables that you may think you don't like.

1 litre chicken or vegetable stock
1 small carrot, grated
280g fresh spinach, coarsely chopped
55g butter
1 onion, chopped
8 garlic cloves, crushed
30g plain flour
250ml skimmed milk
salt and freshly ground black pepper
a pinch of freshly grated nutmeg

1. Put the stock and carrot in a large pan over high heat and bring to the boil. Reduce the heat and simmer for 5 minutes. Stir in the spinach and remove from the heat.

2. Heat the butter in a small non-stick frying pan over medium-high heat, and fry the onion and garlic for 5–10 minutes until the onion is soft. Add the flour, then cook, stirring, over low heat for 3–5 minutes until it forms a paste. Now slowly add the milk, stirring, to make a thick and creamy sauce. Pour this into the stock mixture.

3. Purée the mixture in a blender or food processor until smooth. You may need to do this in batches. Return the mixture to the pan and season with salt, pepper and nutmeg, then heat thoroughly before serving.

Hot Black-Eyed Bean and Chicken Soup

....

Preparation time: **10 minutes** | Cooking time: **40–45 minutes**
Serves **4** | Protein per serving towards DPR: **115g**

This easy soup is spicy and sustaining. It is also very easy to make.

Protein: 460g cooked skinless chicken breasts, diced, adjust
　　to your DPR
225g dried black-eyed beans, soaked overnight and drained
360–480ml chicken or vegetable stock
oil spray
1 celery stick, finely chopped
1 onion, finely chopped
1 carrot, finely chopped
½ red pepper, seeded and finely chopped
4–5 garlic cloves, to taste, crushed
1 bay leaf
½ tsp salt
½ tsp crushed chilli flakes
1 tbsp seasoning mix
freshly ground black pepper
1 tbsp low-fat crème fraîche, to garnish (optional)
4 tbsp chopped fresh tomatoes

1. Put the black-eyed beans and stock in a medium pan over medium heat and bring to the boil. Reduce the heat and simmer for 25–30 minutes until the beans start to become tender.

2. Spray a frying pan with oil spray and add the celery, onion, carrots, pepper and garlic. Cook over medium heat for 3–4 minutes until fragrant and beginning to soften. Add to the beans, along with the remaining ingredients, except the crème fraîche and tomatoes. Simmer for 15 minutes or until the vegetables are soft. Serve with the crème fraîche and tomatoes.

Carrot Soup
with North African Spices

....

Preparation time: **15 minutes** | Cooking time: **30 minutes**
Serves 4

The freshness of carrot and ginger goes well with earthy cumin and coriander, and the sweet potato adds extra creaminess.

1½ tsp cumin seeds
1 tsp coriander seeds
1 tsp crushed chilli flakes (optional)
1 tbsp olive oil
1 onion, thinly sliced
1½ tsp salt
4 small garlic cloves, crushed
3 tsp fresh root ginger, grated, or ½ tsp ground ginger
900g carrots, thinly sliced
1 small sweet potato, thinly sliced
1.2 litres vegetable stock
120ml orange juice (freshly squeezed or from a carton)
1 tsp chopped fresh coriander, to garnish

1. Put the cumin and coriander seeds in a small pan with the chilli flakes, if using, and toast, shaking the pan constantly, for 1 minute or until fragrant. Grind in a spice mill or using a mortar and pestle.

2. Heat the olive oil in a large pan over medium-high heat and add the onion and ½ tsp of the salt. Reduce the heat to medium and fry the onion for 5 minutes or until it begins to soften, then add the garlic, ground spices and ginger. Cook for 10 minutes or until the onion is very soft.

3. Add the carrots, sweet potato, 1 tsp salt and 1 litre of the vegetable stock. Bring to the boil, then reduce the heat, cover and simmer for 15 minutes or until the carrots are very tender.

4. Put the soup in a blender or food processor and purée until smooth, adding extra stock if needed. Return the soup to the pan, add the orange juice and the remaining vegetable stock. Garnish each serving with a sprinkle of fresh coriander and serve.

Thai Chicken Noodle Soup

Preparation time: **10 minutes** | Cooking time: **20 minutes**
Serves **4** | Protein per serving towards DPR: **115g**

Soup is always a hit, and this Thai soup has tantalising aromas of fresh lemongrass. It's the magic potion for a cool evening.

Protein: 460g skinless chicken breasts, cubed, adjust to your DPR
225–280g wide Thai rice noodles
1.5 litres chicken stock
2 lemongrass stalks, finely chopped (or 4 tbsp lemongrass paste from a jar)
2.5cm piece fresh root ginger, peeled and grated
2 carrots, sliced
180g broccoli, cut into florets
140g pak choi, chopped
200ml light coconut milk
4 tbsp soy sauce
1 tbsp hot chilli sauce
oil spray
1 handful of fresh basil, roughly chopped

1. Bring a large pan of water to the boil and add the noodles. Remove from the heat to allow the noodles to soften while you prepare the stock. In another pan over high heat, add the stock, lemongrass, ginger and carrots. Bring to the boil, then add the broccoli and pak choi. Reduce the heat to medium and simmer for 5 minutes or until the vegetables have softened but are still bright in colour. Reduce the heat to low and add the coconut milk, soy sauce and chilli sauce.

2. Heat a medium frying pan coated with oil spray over medium-high heat and cook the cubes of chicken until cooked through. Add the chicken to the pan with the stock.

3. Drain the noodles and divide among soup bowls. Pour several ladles of soup over each bowl of noodles. Sprinkle with fresh basil to serve.

PASTA AND PIZZA

Spaghetti and Meat Sauce

....

Preparation time: **5 minutes** | Cooking time: **15–20 minutes**
Serves **4** | Protein per serving towards DPR: **225g**

This hearty dish will take you back to your youth. Yummy pasta and meat sauce is comfort food at its best.

> Protein: 900g lean minced beef, adjust to your DPR
> 1 tbsp olive oil
> 1 onion, finely chopped
> 3 garlic cloves, crushed
> 450g wholewheat spaghetti, broken into thirds
> 400g can chopped tomatoes
> 400g jar pasta or marinara sauce
> 1 tsp dried oregano
> ¼–½ tsp crushed chilli flakes, to taste
> salt and freshly ground black pepper

1. Heat the oil in a large frying pan over medium-high heat and fry the onion and garlic until soft. Add the minced beef and cook, stirring occasionally, until cooked through.

2. Meanwhile, cook the spaghetti according to the pack instructions. Drain. Return it to the pan and add the tomatoes, pasta sauce, oregano and chilli flakes. Season with salt and pepper. Heat through over medium heat and serve, sprinkled with the Parmesan.

Pasta with Chicken and Fresh Summer Vegetables

....

Preparation time: **15 minutes** | Cooking time: **11 minutes**
Serves **6** | Protein per serving towards DPR: **115g**

Nothing beats freshness like summer vegetables. Be creative in this dish and mix and match your own favourites.

Protein: 690g skinless chicken breast, diced, adjust to
  your DPR
450g wholewheat spaghetti
1 tbsp olive oil
1 small onion, finely chopped
1 garlic clove, crushed
1 yellow pepper, thinly sliced
4 small courgettes, diced
1 bunch of asparagus, woody ends removed, spears cut into
  2.5cm pieces
450g baby plum tomatoes, halved
4 fresh basil leaves, torn
salt and freshly ground black pepper

1. Cook the pasta according to the pack instructions, then drain. Meanwhile, heat the olive oil in a large frying pan over medium heat and fry the chicken and onion until the chicken is cooked through and the onion begins to soften. Add the garlic and fry for 5 minutes.

2. Add the pepper, courgettes and asparagus, and fry until heated through but not completely cooked (you want the vegetables to have a slight crunch).

3. Remove from the heat and add the tomatoes, the pasta and the basil. Season with salt and pepper.

Spicy 'Pepperoni' Pizza

....

Preparation time: **20 minutes** | Cooking time: **17 minutes**
Serves **4** | Protein per serving towards DPR: **115g**

This novel minced-chicken topping is a great way of satisfying any cravings for a spicy pepperoni pizza – without all the fat.

> Protein: 460g chicken breast meat, chopped, adjust to
>   your DPR
> 280g prepared wholemeal pizza base
> ½ tsp fennel seeds
> ¼ onion, halved
> 1 garlic clove
> ¼ tsp crushed chilli flakes
> ¼ tsp freshly ground black pepper
> oil spray
> 240ml low-fat pizza sauce from a jar or passata
> 75g black olives, sliced
> 65g low-fat mozzarella cheese, thinly sliced

1. Preheat the oven to 230°C/450°F/Gas 8. Put the pizza base on a baking sheet or pizza stone and set aside.

2. Heat a large frying pan over medium-high heat, and toast the fennel seeds, shaking the pan constantly, for 1 minute or until just lightly browned. Put the onion and garlic in a food processor and pulse until just chopped. Then add the chicken, fennel seeds, chilli flakes and pepper, and pulse until the mixture is ground.

3. Spray the frying pan with oil spray and brown the chicken mixture over medium heat for 7–10 minutes until cooked through.

4. Spread the pizza sauce onto the pizza base. Top with the chicken mixture, olives and cheese, and bake for 7–10 minutes until the cheese is bubbly and the base is browned.

Spicy Peanut Noodles

Preparation time: **15 minutes** | Cooking time: **30 minutes**
Serves **6**

Plain old pasta gets an Asian twist in this dish that is full of fresh, colourful vegetables. This is great served with salmon.

225g wholewheat linguine
90g reduced-fat smooth peanut butter, no added sugar
2 tbsp soy sauce or tamari
1½ tbsp rice wine vinegar
1–2 tsp hot chilli sauce, to taste
½ tsp sugar
1 red pepper, seeded and cut into thin strips
40g cucumber, sliced
3 spring onions, sliced diagonally into 5mm pieces
2 tbsp chopped fresh coriander or parsley
6 lime wedges

1. Cook the linguine according to the pack instructions, then drain. In a large bowl, add the peanut butter, 50ml water, the soy sauce, vinegar, chilli sauce and sugar, and whisk until blended. The sauce should be creamy; thin it with a little water if needed.

2. Add the linguine, red pepper, cucumber and spring onions, and toss well. Sprinkle with fresh coriander and serve with lime wedges.

Chicken, Spinach and Basil Pizza

....

Preparation time: **15 minutes** | Cooking time: **10 minutes**
Serves **4** | Protein per serving towards DPR: **115g**

Nothing is as satisfying as pizza after a long day at work. Serve with a voluminous side salad and a glass of wine.

Protein: 4 x 115g skinless chicken breasts, diced, adjust to
   your DPR
2 tbsp extra virgin olive oil
2 shallots, finely chopped
4–5 garlic cloves, to taste, crushed
salt and freshly ground black pepper
1 pack pre-prepared wholemeal pizza dough
1 large bunch of fresh basil, finely chopped
1 large handful of fresh baby spinach, finely chopped
175g low-fat hard mozzarella cheese, grated

1. Preheat the oven to 240°C/475°F/Gas 9. Heat 1 tbsp of the oil in a medium frying pan over medium heat and fry the chicken, shallots and garlic. Season with salt and pepper. When cooked through, remove from the heat and set aside.

2. Roll out the dough to a 30–40cm circle, depending on how thin you like your base, and brush the top with the remaining olive oil. Spread the chicken mixture evenly over the dough. Cover with the basil leaves and spinach, and top with the grated cheese. Bake at for about 10 minutes or until the cheese bubbles and the edges of the pizza base are golden brown.

POULTRY

Cashew Chicken Salad with Coriander Dressing

....

Preparation time: **10 minutes** | Cooking time: **5 minutes**
Serves **1** | Protein per serving towards DPR: **115g**

Another quick-cook meal you can whip up in minutes, this filling salad is ideal for lunch or dinner.

Protein: 115g skinless chicken breast, cut into strips, adjust
to your DPR
oil spray
15g sunflower seeds
1 bunch of fresh coriander, leaves chopped
juice of 1–2 oranges
225g mixed salad leaves, such as rocket and baby spinach
2 tbsp cashew nuts
1 small tomato, seeded and diced
¼ avocado, stoned, peeled and sliced
¼ red onion, thinly sliced
55g carrots, grated

1. Heat a small frying pan coated with oil spray over medium heat and fry the chicken strips for 4–6 minutes until completely cooked through. Remove from the frying pan and set aside.

2. In a small bowl, whisk together the sunflower seeds, chopped coriander and orange juice to make the dressing.

3. In a large bowl, toss together the mixed leaves, cashew nuts and coriander dressing until the leaves are coated well. Serve the leaves topped with the chicken, tomato, avocado, red onion and grated carrots.

Red Kidney Bean and Chicken Chilli

....

Preparation time: **10 minutes** | Cooking time: **20 minutes**
Serves **4** | Protein per serving towards DPR: **225g**

For more zing, add a few crushed chilli flakes.

Protein: 900g skinless chicken breasts, cut into 2.5cm pieces,
  adjust to your DPR
oil spray
1 large red pepper, seeded and coarsely diced
1 large onion, chopped
2 red chillies, or to taste, finely chopped
2 garlic cloves, crushed
2½ tbsp plain flour
550ml fat-free, low-salt chicken stock
400g can red kidney beans, drained and rinsed
400g can chopped tomatoes
1 tbsp ground cumin
½ tsp each dried basil, oregano and thyme
1 tbsp low-fat crème fraîche
1 large avocado, stoned, peeled and diced

1. Spray a large frying pan with oil spray. Cook the chicken pieces
   over medium-high heat for 4–5 minutes until browned, then
   remove from the pan and set aside.

2. Add more oil spray and fry the red pepper, onion, chillies and
   garlic, stirring occasionally, for 5 minutes or until tender.

3. Add the flour and stir for 1 minute until thick, then add the
   stock, chicken, beans, tomatoes, cumin, basil, oregano and
   thyme. Bring to the boil over medium-high heat, then reduce
   the heat, cover and simmer until the chicken is cooked through
   and the vegetables are tender. Remove from the heat. Stir in
   the crème fraîche and serve garnished with avocado.

Chicken and Veggie Stir-Fry

....

Preparation time: **10 minutes** | Cooking time: **15 minutes**
Serves **4** | Protein per serving towards DPR: **225g**

Everybody loves a stir-fry; you'll love how simple this one is to make.

> Protein: 900g skinless chicken breast, cut into 1cm cubes,
>   adjust to your DPR
> 3 tbsp olive oil
> 5cm fresh root ginger, or to taste, peeled and grated
> 3 garlic cloves, crushed
> 450g fresh shiitake mushrooms, caps sliced
> 180g broccoli, cut into florets
> 2 red peppers, seeded and sliced
> 2 bunches of spring onions, sliced
> 120ml dry white wine
> 50ml soy sauce
> 1 tbsp toasted sesame oil
> salt and freshly ground black pepper

1. Heat 1½ tbsp olive oil in a large non-stick frying pan or wok over high heat. Add the cubed chicken and fry until no longer pink. Stir gently for 4 minutes or until it begins to brown around the edges. Remove from the pan and set aside.

2. Add the remaining oil to the pan and add the ginger and garlic. Stir-fry for 1 minute. Add the mushrooms and stir-fry for 5 minutes or until tender. Add the broccoli, peppers and spring onions, and stir-fry for 3 minutes or until the vegetables are crisp-tender.

3. Return the chicken to the pan and stir to mix in with the vegetables. In a small bowl, stir together the white wine, soy sauce and sesame oil, then add to the chicken mixture. Heat through for 1 minute. Season with salt and pepper, if you like.

Baked Chicken Burritos

....

Preparation time: **15 minutes** | Cooking time: **20 minutes**
Serves **8** | Protein per serving towards DPR: **115g**

These burritos are low in fat and crunchy on the inside with a crispy, flaky outside. It's a useful meal for busy nights.

Protein: 920g skinless chicken breast, cut into strips, adjust to your DPR
40g pine nuts
30g pumpkin seeds
1 tbsp extra virgin olive oil
2 onions, chopped
1 red pepper, seeded and chopped
2–3 garlic cloves, to taste, crushed
370g tomato sauce from a jar
1 tbsp chilli powder
1–2 tsp ground cumin, to taste
1 tsp dried oregano
1 tsp dried basil
1 tsp salt
½ tsp freshly ground black pepper
140g frozen sweetcorn
30g stoned black olives (optional)
oil spray
8 wholemeal tortillas or chapattis
55g low-fat mild Cheddar cheese, grated
1 tbsp guacamole (optional)
1 tbsp low-fat crème fraîche (optional)
unlimited fat-free salsa (optional)

1. Preheat the oven to 180°C/350°F/Gas 4. Put the pine nuts and pumpkin seeds in a pan and toast over medium heat, shaking the pan constantly, for 2 minutes or until golden. Remove from the pan and set aside.

2. Heat the olive oil in a large non-stick frying pan over medium heat and fry the chicken, onions, red pepper and garlic until the onion is golden. Add the tomato sauce to the pan with the chilli powder, cumin, oregano, basil, salt, pepper, sweetcorn and olives, if using. Add the pine nuts and pumpkin seeds and cook, stirring frequently, until the mixture begins to boil. Remove from the heat.

3. Coat a 23 x 33cm ovenproof dish lightly with oil spray. Put one tortilla on the work surface and spread one-eighth of the mixture over it. Roll it up, wrapping it tightly and put it seam-side down in the pan. Repeat until all the tortillas are filled.

4. Bake the burritos uncovered for 15 minutes or until crisp. Top with grated cheese and bake for a further 5 minutes until the cheese has melted. Serve the burritos with guacamole, crème fraîche and salsa.

Extra-healthy Spinach Salad with Turkey

....

Preparation time: **10 minutes** | Cooking time: **20 minutes**
Serves **8** | Protein per serving towards DPR: **115g**

This generous salad is tasty enough to please the entire family.

Protein: 920g turkey breast, cubed, adjust to your DPR
1 medium egg
30g plain flour
3 tsp garlic powder
1 tsp onion powder
½ tsp freshly ground black pepper
3 tbsp plus 120ml extra virgin olive oil
120ml white wine vinegar
50g caster sugar
3 tbsp orange juice
85g baby spinach
85g mixed salad leaves
400g can mandarin oranges, drained
55g walnuts, chopped
75g dried cranberries
1 red pepper, seeded and sliced
75g feta cheese, crumbled (optional)

1. Beat the egg in a small bowl. In another small bowl, mix together the flour, garlic and onion powders and black pepper. Dip the turkey cubes in the egg and dust with the flour mixture.

2. Heat the 3 tbsp oil in a large frying pan over medium-high heat. Fry the turkey cubes for 10 minutes, turning, so that they are golden and crispy on all sides. Remove from the pan and leave to cool. In a small pan, combine the 120ml olive oil

with the white wine vinegar, sugar and orange juice and cook over medium heat for 2–3 minutes until the sugar dissolves, to make a dressing. Transfer to a bowl and leave to cool.

3. Put the spinach in a large serving bowl and add the salad leaves, mandarin oranges, walnuts, cranberries and red pepper. Add half the dressing, toss well and divide among 8 individual bowls. Top with the turkey cubes and feta cheese, and drizzle the remaining dressing evenly over.

Puy Lentil Salad

Preparation time: **5 minutes** | Cooking time: **20 minutes**
Serves **5** | Protein per serving towards DPR: **10g**

Puy lentils and bacon is a classic combination. This recipe uses turkey rashers instead, to give a hint of bacon without all the extra fat and calories. If turkey rashers are unavailable, use 50g Serrano ham – simply chop and stir through the cooled lentil mixture.

Protein: 2 turkey rashers, adjust to your DPR
200g dried Puy lentils
800ml vegetable stock
5 halves sun-dried tomatoes
2 tbsp walnut pieces
2 tsp olive oil
freshly ground black pepper

1. Rinse the lentils then put in a pan, cover with the stock and simmer until cooked, about 25–30 minutes. Drain and place in a bowl to cool.

2. Grill the turkey rashers until crispy. Transfer to kitchen paper to drain and cool, then chop or crumble.

3. Cover the sun-dried tomatoes in hot water, remove and blot with kitchen paper to remove excess oil. Chop the tomatoes and add to the lentils, along with turkey, walnut pieces and oil. Stir well and add pepper to taste.

Shepherd's Pie with Chicken

....

Preparation time: **20 minutes** | Cooking time: **1 hour**
Serves **8** | Protein per serving towards DPR: **55g**

You're in for a real treat with this version of the family favourite.

Protein: 440g skinless chicken breast, cubed, adjust to
   your DPR
oil spray
1 onion, thinly sliced
65g green beans, cut into 2.5cm pieces
1 small courgette, halved lengthways and sliced
1 large carrot, sliced
1 large parsnip, sliced
65g frozen peas, thawed
100g mushrooms, sliced

Mashed potatoes
4 large all-purpose potatoes, such as Maris Piper, unpeeled
   and scrubbed
3 tbsp butter
½ tsp coarsely ground black pepper

Gravy
35g plain wholemeal flour
350ml hot vegetable stock
2 tbsp tamari
2 tbsp nutritional yeast flakes (not baker's or brewer's yeast)
salt and freshly ground black pepper

1. Preheat the oven to 190°C/375°F/Gas 5. Heat a medium frying pan over medium-high heat, spray with oil, add the chicken and onion and fry until the chicken is cooked through, then set aside.

2. To make the mashed potatoes, cook the potatoes in a large pan of boiling water for 20 minutes or until tender. While the potatoes are cooking, steam the remaining vegetables for 5 minutes or until they are just beginning to soften. Set aside. Drain and mash the potatoes, then add the butter and pepper.

3. To make the gravy, heat a heavy frying pan over medium heat, then add the flour and stir continuously with a wooden spoon until it turns a rich brown colour. Very slowly add the hot vegetable stock and tamari, stirring constantly, until completely smooth, then cook for 5 minutes. Stir in the nutritional yeast, salt and pepper. Mix in the chicken and vegetables and transfer to an ovenproof dish. Pour over the gravy and mix well. Cover with the mashed potatoes and bake for 40 minutes or until golden brown.

Indian Spiced Chicken

....

Preparation time: **10 minutes** | Cooking time: **20 minutes**
Serves **2** | Protein per serving towards DPR: **225g**

Cumin, coriander, mint, turmeric and ginger gives baked chicken plenty of flavour.

> Protein: 2 x 225g skinless chicken breasts, adjust to your DPR
> 1 tsp curry powder
> ½ tsp salt
> ½ tsp crushed chilli flakes
> 1 tsp ground cumin
> 1 tsp ground coriander
> 1 tsp dried mint
> ½ tsp turmeric
> ½ tsp ground ginger
> oil spray

1. Preheat the oven to 180°C/350°F/Gas 4. Put the curry powder in a small bowl and add the salt, crushed chilli flakes, cumin, coriander, mint, turmeric and ginger. Mix together well.

2. Spray each side of the chicken breasts with oil spray, then sprinkle with the spice mix. Put into an ovenproof dish and bake for 15–20 minutes until the chicken is no longer pink.

Zesty Broccoli Coleslaw Salad with Chicken

....

Preparation time: **15–20 minutes**
Serves **4** | Protein per serving towards DPR: **225g**

Another no-cook meal! Just toss it all together for a super easy, tasty dish.

Protein: 900g cooked chicken mini fillets, adjust to your DPR
225g broccoli, thinly sliced, or coarsely grated
225g carrots, coarsely grated
1 small red pepper, seeded and thinly sliced
5 tbsp chopped fresh coriander
2 spring onions, chopped
5 tbsp roasted peanuts, chopped

Dressing
2 tbsp toasted sesame oil
1 tbsp rice vinegar
1 tbsp balsamic vinegar
1 tsp hot chilli sauce
1 tsp agave nectar

1. To make the dressing, in a small bowl, whisk together the sesame oil, vinegars, chilli sauce and agave nectar.

2. In a large bowl, toss together the broccoli, carrots, red pepper, chicken, fresh coriander, spring onions and dressing. Top with chopped peanuts and serve.

Spicy Chicken and Cannellini Bean Chilli

....

Preparation time: **20 minutes** | Cooking time: **20 minutes**
Serves **4** | Protein per serving towards DPR: **115g**

High in protein and fibre – a spicy chilli to keep you going for hours.

> Protein: 460g skinless chicken breast, cut into 2.5cm pieces,
>   adjust to your DPR
> oil spray
> 1 red pepper, seeded and chopped
> 1 large onion, chopped
> 1 chilli, seeded and finely chopped
> 2–3 garlic cloves, crushed
> 3 tbsp plain flour
> 550ml low-salt, fat-free chicken stock
> 1½ x 400g cans cannellini beans, drained and rinsed
> 1 tbsp ground cumin
> a pinch of crushed chilli flakes or cayenne pepper
> 2 tbsp low-fat crème fraîche
> juice of 1 lime
> 1 avocado, stoned, peeled and sliced

1. Spray a large frying pan with oil spray and heat over medium-high heat. Fry the chicken pieces for 5 minutes or until brown. Transfer to a plate.

2. Spray the same frying pan with additional oil spray and fry the pepper, onion, chilli and garlic over medium-high heat until tender. Add the flour, stirring quickly, and cook for 1 minute. Stir in the stock, chicken, beans, cumin and crushed chilli flakes. Bring to boiling over high heat. Reduce the heat to low and simmer for 10 minutes or until the chicken is no longer pink and the vegetables are tender. Remove from the heat.

3. Stir in the crème fraîche and then add the lime juice. Spoon into 4 serving bowls and top each bowl with a quarter of the avocado slices.

Thai Chicken Salad

....

Preparation time: **10 minutes**
Serves **4** | Protein per serving towards DPR: **115g**

No cooking required for this protein-rich Thai sensation!

Protein: 460g cooked skinless chicken breasts, cut into 2.5cm pieces, adjust to your DPR
½ lettuce, leaves sliced
¼ cucumber, diced
180g tomatoes, seeded and diced
1 bunch of spring onions, sliced
40g dry-roasted peanuts, chopped

Dressing
250ml fat-free, low-salt chicken stock
2 tbsp smooth peanut butter, no added sugar
250ml soy sauce
1 tsp lime zest
2 tbsp lime juice
2 tsp toasted sesame oil

1. Divide the lettuce among 4 individual plates. Top with the chicken, cucumber, tomatoes and spring onions.

2. To make the dressing, in a small bowl whisk together the stock, peanut butter, soy sauce, lime zest and juice, and toasted sesame oil. Drizzle the dressing over the salad. Top with the peanuts.

BEEF AND PORK

Spicy Meatballs

....

Preparation time: **10 minutes** | Cooking time: **15 minutes**
Serves **4** | Protein per serving towards DPR: **115g**

These meatballs are easy to make and are a real treat stuffed in a pitta with salad for lunch. They also taste great cold in a pitta if you need to take your lunch with you to eat on the run.

> Protein: 460g extra lean ground beef, adjust to your DPR
> 1 garlic clove, crushed
> 1 onion, very finely chopped or grated
> ½ tsp dried crushed chillies
> 1 tsp garam masala
> salt and freshly ground pepper

1. Put all the ingredients in a bowl and mix thoroughly, until the mixture holds together. Divide the mixture into pieces roughly the size of golf balls and roll into balls between your palms.

2. Put the meatballs in a baking tray and bake in a 190°C/375°F/ Gas 5 oven for 15–20 minutes until cooked through.

Beefy Mushroom Burgers

....

Preparation time: **15 minutes** | Cooking time: **16–20 minutes**
Serves **4** | Protein per serving towards DPR: **115g**

You can enjoy our Overnight Diet burger – and still lose weight!

Protein: 460g lean minced beef, adjust to your DPR
25g dried porcini or shiitake mushrooms, finely chopped
   (no need to soak)
2 tsp Worcestershire sauce
salt and freshly ground black pepper
225g button, chestnut or shiitake mushrooms, sliced
1 large onion, thinly sliced
2 tbsp olive oil
4 wholemeal burger buns
lettuce, tomatoes and pickles, to serve (optional)

1. Put the chopped dried mushrooms in a large bowl and add the minced beef, Worcestershire sauce, and salt and pepper, then thoroughly mix together (use your hands to get a better mixture). Shape the mixture into 4 burgers and, using your thumb, make an indentation in the centre of each.

2. Heat the grill to high. Heat a large heavy-based frying pan over high heat for 1 minute. Add the fresh mushrooms to the pan and dry-fry them for 2–3 minutes until they release their liquid. Add the onion and the olive oil, then stir to combine and continue to fry over high heat for 1 minute. Season with salt and cook until the onions soften and begin to brown. Turn off the heat and transfer the vegetables to a bowl.

3. Grill the burgers according to your preference – between 5 and 8 minutes per side. Put a grilled burger onto the bottom half of each burger bun, then top with the mushrooms and onions. Add lettuce, tomatoes and pickles to serve.

Braised Fillet Steak in Mushroom and Red Wine Sauce

....

Preparation time: **15 minutes** | Cooking time: **12–18 minutes**
Serves **2** | Protein per serving towards DPR: **225g**

Steak and mushrooms are another all-time favourite. Try it with quinoa and a large side salad for a twist.

Protein: 2 x 225g fillet steaks, adjust to your DPR
1 tbsp plus 1 tsp plain flour
1 tbsp olive oil
115g chestnut mushrooms, sliced
½ onion, finely chopped
2 garlic cloves, crushed
120ml dry red wine
1 tsp Dijon or spicy brown mustard
½ tsp dried thyme
salt and freshly ground black pepper
120ml vegetable stock
4 tbsp chopped fresh parsley, to garnish

1. Coat the fillet steak pieces in the 1 tbsp flour. Heat the oil in a large pan over medium-high heat. Add the fillet steaks when the oil is hot and cook for 1–2 minutes on each side. Remove the steaks from the frying pan and cover to keep warm.

2. Add the mushrooms, onion and garlic to the pan and fry for 7–10 minutes until softened and lightly browned. In a small bowl, whisk together the red wine, mustard and thyme, then add it to the mushroom mixture. Season with salt and pepper and cook for a further 2–3 minutes until the sauce is slightly thickened. Whisk together the 1 tsp flour and the vegetable stock, then add to the mushroom mixture. Simmer for 2–3 minutes, or until thickened, stirring constantly. Serve the steaks with the mushroom sauce, garnished with chopped parsley.

Old-fashioned Beef Stew

....

Preparation time: **30 minutes** | Cooking time: **1½ hours**
Serves **12** | Protein per serving towards DPR: **225g**

This hearty beef stew is reminiscent of good home cooking from the past. Pair it with a colourful salad to meet all your nutrient needs. It freezes well so you will have plenty for those days when you need something fast.

Protein: 2.7kg chuck or braising steak, cut into 5cm pieces, adjust to your DPR
3 tbsp olive oil
2 tsp salt
1 tbsp freshly ground black pepper
2 onions, quartered
30g plain flour
3 garlic cloves, crushed
250ml dry red wine
750ml beef stock
½ tsp dried rosemary
1 bay leaf
½ tsp dried thyme
1 large King Edward potato, unpeeled, cut into small cubes
6 carrots, cut into 1cm slices
2 celery sticks, cut into 1cm slices
fresh parsley, to garnish (optional)

1. Heat the olive oil in a large, heavy-based flameproof casserole or pan over medium-high heat. Add the beef and brown well on all sides. Stir in the salt and pepper, then remove the beef using a slotted spoon. Set aside.

2. Add the onions to the casserole and fry for 5 minutes or until softened. Reduce the heat to medium-low, add the flour and cook for 2 minutes, stirring frequently, until thickened. Add the garlic and cook for 1 minute.

3. Pour in the wine to deglaze the casserole, scraping any brown pieces stuck to the base using a spatula. The flour will start to thicken the wine as it comes to a simmer. Simmer for 5 minutes, then add the stock, rosemary, bay leaf, thyme and the beef. Bring back to the boil then turn down to a gentle simmer. Cover and cook over very low heat for 1 hour.

4. Add the potato, carrots and celery, and simmer, covered, for another 30 minutes or until the meat and vegetables are tender. Remove from the heat and leave to stand for 15 minutes, covered tightly. Garnish with the fresh parsley, if you like.

Vegetable Stir-fry (with beef or pork)

....

Preparation time: **5–8 minutes** | Cooking time: **8–10 minutes**
Serves **4** | Protein per serving towards DPR: **115g**

Broccoli, cauliflower, sugar snap peas and carrots add sparkles of dazzling colour as well as calcium to this stir-fry. Add flavoursome beef or pork to round out the meal.

> Protein: 460g lean beef or pork, cut into cubes, adjust to your DPR
> 2 garlic cloves, crushed
> 2.5cm piece fresh root ginger, peeled and grated
> 2 tbsp hoisin sauce
> 1 tbsp extra virgin olive oil
> 225g cauliflower, cut into florets
> 65g sugar snap peas
> 1 large carrot, thinly sliced
> 1 onion, thinly sliced
> 180g broccoli, cut into florets
> 1½ tsp cornflour
> 3 tbsp dry cooking sherry or rice wine vinegar

1. Combine the garlic, ginger and hoisin sauce in a small bowl and set aside. Heat the oil in a large heavy-based frying pan or wok (with a lid) over medium-high heat and fry the beef or pork until almost cooked through.

2. Add the cauliflower, sugar snap peas, carrot and onion. Stir-fry for 4–5 minutes, then add the broccoli and 2 tbsp water. Cover and cook for 4–5 minutes until the vegetables are tender but still crisp. Combine the cornflour with 120ml cold water in a small bowl. Add the ginger sauce to the stir-fry with the sherry and cornflour mixture, and stir until the sauce is thickened.

Pork Escalopes with Caribbean Salsa

....

Preparation time: **8 minutes** | Cooking time: **6 minutes**
Serves **2** | Protein per serving towards DPR: **225g**

This delicious yet simple recipe has a refreshing taste that goes well with green vegetables.

Protein: 450g pork leg escalopes, adjust to your DPR
227g can pineapple pieces in juice, drained
1 small mango, peeled, stoned and chopped
juice of ½ lime
2 tbsp chopped fresh coriander

1. Grill the pork escalopes under a medium grill for about 3 minutes each side, or until no longer pink.

2. Mix the remaining ingredients in a bowl and serve alongside the pork.

Rosemary Roast Pork

....

Preparation time: **10 minutes** | Cooking time: **2 hours**
Serves **6** | Protein per serving towards DPR: **225g**

Roast pork doesn't have to be complicated to cook – this one is simple and succulent. You won't be disappointed.

> Protein: 1.3kg pork tenderloin, adjust to your DPR
> 1 tbsp plus 2 tsp olive oil
> 4–8 garlic cloves, halved
> 3 tbsp dried rosemary, chopped

1. Preheat the oven to 190°C/375°F/Gas 5. Pour the 1 tbsp olive oil into a large, heavy-based casserole and add the pork tenderloin. Rub the tenderloin liberally with the 2 tsp olive oil, then lay the garlic halves on top. Sprinkle with the rosemary.

2. Cover and cook in the oven for 2 hours, or until tender and cooked through (or the internal temperature of the pork reaches 160°C). Alternatively, you can use a slow-cooker. Put the prepared tenderloin into the slow-cooker and add 250–450ml water to come to at least 2.5cm up the meat. Cover and cook on low heat for 8–9 hours until the meat is tender and can be pulled apart with a fork.

SEAFOOD

Apple Tuna Wrap

....

Preparation time: **2–4 minutes** | Cooking time: **5–6 minutes**
Serves **3** | Protein per serving towards DPR: **115g**

This recipe takes the typical tuna sandwich in a tasty new and healthy direction.

> Protein: 2 x 185g cans tuna chunks in water, drained, adjust to
> your DPR
> 60g fat-free Greek yogurt
> 1 small apple, cored and chopped
> 1 tsp Dijon mustard
> 1 tsp honey or agave nectar
> 3 wholemeal wraps
> 2 large handfuls of mixed salad leaves
> 1 tomato, seeded and diced
> 1 large carrot, grated
> 1 beetroot, grated
> 100g alfalfa sprouts
> fruit, to serve

In a small bowl, mix together the tuna, yogurt, apple, mustard and honey. Divide among the wholemeal wraps. Top with salad leaves, tomato, grated carrot, grated beetroot and alfalfa. Roll up and serve with fruit.

Crusty Oven-fried Fish

....

Preparation time: **10 minutes** | Cooking time: **8 minutes**
Serves **4** | Protein per serving towards DPR: **225g**

Love fish but not sure how to cook it? This oven-fried fish is as easy as it gets.

Protein: 4 x 225g pieces cod 2–2.5cm thick, adjust to your DPR
75g plain dried breadcrumbs
90g polenta
2 tbsp finely grated Parmesan cheese
1 tsp salt
¼ tsp black pepper
¼ tsp chilli powder
1 egg and 2 egg whites, lightly beaten
3 tbsp olive oil

1. Preheat the oven to 240°C/475°F/Gas 9. Put the breadcrumbs in a large plastic bag and add the polenta, Parmesan cheese, salt, pepper and chilli powder. Shake to mix thoroughly.

2. Put the fish pieces into the plastic bag one at a time and shake to coat. Dip the fish into the beaten egg and drop into the plastic bag for a second coating of crumb mixture.

3. Line a baking sheet with baking parchment or foil and brush with the olive oil. Put the breaded fish onto the baking sheet and cook in the oven for 4 minutes, then flip the fish over and cook for a further 4 minutes until both sides are golden brown and the fish is flaky when pierced with a knife.

Lemon Roasted Salmon

....

Preparation time: **15 minutes, plus 10 minutes** marinating
Cooking time: **15 minutes** | Serves **4** | Protein per serving
towards DPR: **225g**

Choose wild salmon rather than farmed, if you can, for a mild and 'not so fishy' flavour.

Protein: 4 x 225g salmon fillets, adjust to your DPR
1 tsp grated lemon zest
2 tbsp fresh lemon juice
2 tbsp honey
½ tsp salt
½ tsp ground coriander
¼ tsp chilli powder
175g can orange juice concentrate, thawed
oil spray
1 small orange, thinly sliced, to garnish

1. Preheat the oven to 200°C/400°F/Gas 6. In a bowl, whisk together the lemon zest and juice, honey, salt, coriander, chilli powder and orange juice concentrate. Put the fish skin side down in a large shallow dish and pour the citrus mixture over the top. Leave to marinate for 10 minutes.

2. Coat a roasting tin with oil spray, then transfer the fish to the tin. Bake for 15 minutes or until the fish flakes easily with a knife. Garnish with orange slices and serve.

Asian Salad with Tuna

....

Preparation time: **15 minutes** | Cooking time: **5–6 minutes**
Serves **2** | Protein per serving towards DPR: **115g**

The sesame miso dressing takes an ordinary salad and turns it into an inspiring creation.

Protein: 2 x 115g fresh tuna steaks, adjust to your DPR
140g mixed salad leaves
1 small carrot, grated
25g beansprouts

Sesame miso dressing
2 tbsp sesame seeds, plus extra to garnish
75ml rice wine vinegar
50ml white miso
2 tbsp lemon juice
2 tsp grated fresh root ginger
1 tbsp sugar
1 tsp toasted sesame oil
3 tbsp mirin or cooking sake

1. In a small frying pan, toast the sesame seeds for the dressing over high heat, shaking the pan constantly, for 2–3 minutes until the seeds begin to pop. Set aside. Heat a medium heavy-based frying pan over medium-high heat and sear the tuna for 1–2 minutes on each side; the tuna will still be uncooked in the centre. If you prefer, cook the tuna until well done, for 3–4 minutes per side.

2. In a medium mixing bowl, toss together the mixed salad leaves, carrot and beansprouts. Whisk all the dressing ingredients together in a small bowl, then drizzle the dressing over the salad leaves and toss well to coat. Serve the steak on the salad, garnished with a few sesame seeds.

Mediterranean Tuna Salad

....

Preparation time: **10–12 minutes** | Serves **4** | Protein per serving towards DPR: **115g**

Chickpeas provide additional fibre and protein to this salad. Add colourful vegetables for an antioxidant boost.

Protein: 3 x 160g cans tuna in water, drained well, adjust to your DPR
Protein: 1 hardboiled egg, finely diced, adjust to your DPR
½ x 400g can chickpeas, drained and rinsed
1 large red pepper, seeded and finely diced
1 red onion, finely chopped
1 handful of fresh parsley, chopped
4 tsp capers, rinsed
1½ tsp finely chopped fresh rosemary
120ml lemon juice
4 tbsp extra-virgin olive oil
¼ tsp salt
freshly ground black pepper
200g mixed salad leaves

1. Put the chickpeas in a medium bowl and add the tuna, red pepper, onion, parsley, capers, rosemary, 60ml of the lemon juice and 2 tbsp of the oil. Combine well.

2. In a separate large bowl combine the remaining lemon juice and oil with the salt and pepper to taste. Add the salad leaves and toss to coat. Divide the salad among 4 plates. Top each with a quarter of the tuna salad and the hardboiled egg.

Pan-fried
Wild Salmon with Mustard Sauce

....

Preparation time: **10 minutes** | Cooking time: **20 minutes**
Serves **4** | Protein per serving towards DPR: **225g**

*Take a walk on the wild side with spicy salmon fillets. Use wild
salmon if you can.*

> Protein: 4 x 225g salmon fillets, 2.5cm thick, adjust to your
>   DPR
> 1 tbsp olive oil
> freshly ground black pepper
> 120ml vegetable stock
> 2 tbsp balsamic vinegar
> 1 tbsp Dijon or spicy mustard
> 2 tsp dark soft brown sugar

1. Heat the oil in a frying pan over medium heat. Coat the flesh
   side of the salmon with ground black pepper, then put the
   salmon, skin side up, into the hot frying pan and cook for 4
   minutes on each side or until cooked through. (If you like,
   cook for a little less time so that it remains slightly under-
   cooked in the centre.) Remove the salmon to a plate; cover to
   keep warm and set aside.

2. Pour the stock into the frying pan and add the balsamic vinegar, mustard and sugar. Bring to the boil, then simmer over
   medium heat for 10 minutes or until the mixture is slightly
   thickened and has reduced by half. Serve the salmon with the
   sauce poured over.

Tuna Delight

....

Preparation time: **10 minutes** | Serves **4** | Protein per serving towards DPR: **115g**

Tuna salad served with salsa – use an extra-spicy salsa if you want to turn up the heat – it's up to you.

Protein: 3 x 160g cans tuna chunks in water, drained, adjust to your DPR
Protein: 1 hardboiled egg, diced, adjust to your DPR
75g stoned black olives, sliced
1 bunch of spring onions, sliced
1 celery stick, sliced
90g fat-free salsa, plus extra for drizzling (optional)
120g low-fat crème fraîche
1 tsp ground cumin
lettuce leaves, shredded
raw vegetables for serving (such as cauliflower or broccoli florets, red pepper, carrot or celery sticks, raw courgette slices)

1. Put the tuna in a medium bowl and add the olives, spring onions and celery. Mix together well. In a small bowl, combine the salsa, crème fraîche and cumin. Tip the salsa mixture into the bowl with the tuna, add the diced egg and mix well.

2. To serve, put the lettuce onto 4 plates and top with a quarter of the tuna mixture. Add the raw vegetables, then drizzle with extra salsa, if you like, and serve.

VEGETABLES, SIDE DISHES AND SNACKS

Berry, Carrot and Apple Salad

························

Preparation time: **10–15 minutes** | Serves **4**

Looking for a little intensity in your life? You can find it on your plate with this vibrant sweet-and-sour marriage of fruit and vegetables.

2 tbsp fat-free Greek yogurt
juice of 1 lime
2 tbsp extra virgin olive oil
4 tsp white wine vinegar
2 tsp agave nectar
3 handfuls of rocket
1 large carrot, peeled and coarsely grated
½ apple, coarsely grated or cut into thin slices
125g raspberries (or berries of choice)

1. In a small mixing bowl, whisk together the yogurt, lime juice, oil, vinegar and agave nectar. Measure out 2 tbsp and put it into a small bowl.

2. Put the rocket into a bowl and add the carrot and apple, then toss together. Add the larger portion of yogurt dressing and toss well. Divide among 4 plates and top with the berries. Drizzle with the remaining dressing.

Bean, Corn and Quinoa Salad

....

Preparation time: **15 minutes**, plus at least **30 minutes** chilling
Serves **4**

*Fibre-rich, colourful and bursting with dynamic flavour, this salad is
sure to become an all-time favourite.*

270g canned red kidney beans, drained and rinsed
185g cooked quinoa (75g raw weight)
140g frozen sweetcorn, thawed
1 red onion, finely chopped
½ red pepper, seeded and chopped
1 tomato, seeded and chopped
1 tsp salt
1 handful of fresh coriander or parsley, leaves chopped
1 tbsp finely chopped fresh basil leaves
2 tbsp lime or lemon juice
1 tbsp white balsamic vinegar (or apple cider vinegar)

Put all the ingredients in a large bowl and combine well. Chill for
at least 30 minutes before serving.

Fennel, Apple and Rocket Salad

....

Preparation time: **15 minutes**, plus **30 minutes** marinating
Serves **4**

Fresh fennel's crispy crunch has the flavour of anise (liquorice). Paired with crispy green apple and peppery rocket, this salad is anything but ordinary.

1 tbsp white balsamic vinegar
salt and freshly ground black pepper
3 tbsp olive oil
1 tbsp chopped fresh parsley
2 small fennel bulbs
1 green apple
1 tbsp lemon juice
3 handfuls of rocket
25g Parmesan cheese, grated
40g roasted, unsalted almonds

1. In a small bowl, whisk the vinegar with salt and pepper, then gradually whisk in the oil. Add the parsley and set the dressing aside.

2. Using a small, very sharp knife, remove the core at the base of the fennel bulbs and very thinly slice the bulbs. Core and thinly slice the apple and toss the apple with lemon juice. Set aside.

3. In a large bowl, toss together the fennel and apples with half the dressing. Cover tightly and chill for 30 minutes for the flavours to develop.

4. Add the rocket to the fennel mixture and toss gently with the remaining dressing. Arrange on 4 salad plates and sprinkle with the grated cheese and almonds.

Avocado, Fennel and Citrus Salad

....

Preparation time: **20 minutes** | Serves **4**

Light and refreshing, this salad can be paired with beef, poultry or seafood dishes.

1 orange
1 pink grapefruit
3 tbsp white balsamic or red wine vinegar
2 tsp fennel seeds, toasted and crushed
3 tbsp olive oil
salt and freshly ground black pepper
2 large ripe avocados, halved, stoned and peeled
1 fennel bulb, halved and thinly sliced
1 large handful of pea shoots
2 shallots, finely chopped

1. Grate ¼ tsp zest from the orange. Cut off the peel from the orange and grapefruit using a small, sharp knife, then cut the juicy segments away from the white membranes. Work over a small bowl to catch any juice.

2. In the same bowl, make the salad dressing by whisking together the vinegar, fennel seeds, orange zest, 1 tbsp orange juice and 1 tbsp grapefruit juice caught from each fruit. Gradually whisk in the oil. Season with salt and pepper.

3. Put an avocado half onto each serving plate and drizzle 1 tsp of the dressing over each. Put the sliced fennel, pea shoots and shallots in a bowl and toss with enough of the remaining dressing to coat. Generously top the avocado halves with the fennel mixture. Arrange the reserved grapefruit and orange segments around the avocados. Drizzle with more of the dressing and serve.

Celeriac Rémoulade

....

Preparation time: **20 minutes** | Serves **4**

A creamy dressing combined with celeriac makes a side-dish solution for practically any main dish.

450g celeriac
1½ tsp salt
1½ tsp fresh lemon juice

Dressing
60g Dijon mustard
3 tbsp boiling water
75–120ml extra-virgin olive oil
3 tbsp white wine vinegar
3 tbsp chopped fresh parsley
salt and freshly ground white pepper

1. If using a food processor, cut the celeriac into 2.5cm chunks then use the food processor to slice the celeriac chunks into matchsticks. Alternatively, very thinly slice the celeriac and cut into matchsticks. Put the celeriac in a large bowl and immediately toss with the salt and lemon juice to prevent discoloration and to tenderise the celeriac.

2. To make the dressing, put the mustard in a medium bowl and drizzle in the boiling water while whisking continuously, then whisk in enough of the oil, then the vinegar, to make a thick, creamy sauce.

3. Rinse the celeriac in cold water, then drain and dry in a salad spinner or using a clean teatowel. Fold the celeriac into the dressing, add the parsley and season with salt and pepper if needed.

Japanese Spinach Salad

·····················

Preparation time: **15 minutes**, plus **30 minutes** chilling
Cooking time: **2–3 minutes** | Serves **2**

This is a simple and easy vitamin-rich side dish that goes well with main dishes, such as Pan-fried Salmon with Mustard Sauce (page 245). Toasting the sesame seeds enhances the flavour.

450g baby spinach (or 280g frozen spinach)
2 tbsp, plus 1 tsp sesame seeds
1 tsp sugar
4 tsp soy sauce
1 tbsp rice vinegar
½ tsp toasted sesame oil

1. Line a baking sheet with baking parchment. Bring a large pan of salted water to the boil. Fill a medium bowl with ice cubes and water. Add the fresh spinach to the pan and boil for 20 seconds. (If using frozen spinach, put it in a small pan and cook it in just a small amount of water until it falls apart.) Drain the spinach and plunge it into the iced water. After a few seconds, when the spinach has cooled, transfer it to a colander.

2. Using your hands, squeeze out as much of the spinach water as you can, then spread the spinach over the lined baking sheet and cover loosely with kitchen paper or a teatowel. Chill in fridge for 30 minutes.

3. In a small frying pan, toast the 2 tbsp sesame seeds over high heat, shaking the pan constantly, for 2–3 minutes until the seeds begin to pop. Using a spice grinder or mortar and pestle, grind the sesame seeds with ½ tsp of the sugar.

4. In a medium bowl, combine the remaining sugar with the soy sauce, rice vinegar and toasted sesame oil. Add the ground sesame seeds.

5. Add the chilled spinach and toss it with your hands to thoroughly combine with the spice mixture. Sprinkle with the remaining sesame seeds and serve.

Garlic Pitta Chips

Preparation time: **15 minutes** | Cooking time: **10–12 minutes** Serves **6**

Tastier than crisps and better for you, these pitta chips are an ideal complement for soups and salads. Try them with the Hummus and Pesto Soup (page 207).

1½ tbsp olive oil
1 garlic clove, crushed
1 tsp salt
½ tsp freshly ground black pepper
3 wholemeal pitta breads, cut into 4–6 triangles each

1. Preheat the oven to 180°C/350°F/Gas 4. Cover two large baking sheets with foil. Put the olive oil, garlic, salt and pepper in a small food processor or blender and pulse to combine.

2. Open the pitta triangles to separate the tops from the bottoms and put the triangles on the baking sheets. Brush lightly with the olive oil seasoning mixture. Bake for 10–12 minutes or until golden brown. Let the pitta chips cool on the baking sheets before serving.

Spiced Cauliflower Cheese

....

Preparation time: **10–20 minutes** | Cooking time: **40 minutes**
Serves **8**

Traditional cauliflower cheese is given a strong flavour boost to make it extra special. This recipe freezes well so freeze any leftovers for another meal. Eat within 6–8 weeks.

1 large cauliflower, broken into florets
2 tbsp butter
3 tbsp plain flour
475ml skimmed milk
2 garlic cloves, crushed
170g low-fat mature Cheddar cheese, grated
50g Parmesan cheese
½ cup nutritional yeast flakes
¼ tsp chilli powder
½ tsp paprika
1 egg
25g fresh breadcrumbs

1. Preheat the oven to 180°C/350°F/Gas 4 and coat a 33 × 23cm baking dish with oil spray. Boil the cauliflower florets in a large pan of salted water for 5–7 minutes until tender. Drain well and reserve 250ml of the cooking liquid.

2. Using the same pan over medium heat, melt the butter, whisk in the flour, then cook, whisking constantly, for 1 minute. Whisk in the milk, garlic and reserved cooking liquid, then cook for 7–10 minutes until the sauce is thickened, whisking constantly to prevent burning.

3. Remove from the heat and stir in both cheeses, the nutritional yeast, chilli powder, paprika and the egg. Continue

stirring over low heat until the cheese has melted. Fold in the cauliflower.

4. Pour the mixture into the prepared dish and spread evenly. Top with the breadcrumbs and bake for 30 minutes or until hot and bubbly.

Baked Cheesy Tomatoes

Preparation time: **2–4 minutes** | Cooking time: **15 minutes**
Serves **4**

Crispy on top, soft and juicy underneath, these baked tomatoes serve as an impeccable complement to any meal.

   4 tomatoes, halved horizontally
   35g low-fat mature Cheddar cheese, grated
   1 tsp fresh oregano, chopped
   salt and freshly ground black pepper
   4 tsp extra-virgin olive oil

Preheat the oven to 230°C/450°F/Gas 8. Put the tomatoes cut-side up on a baking sheet. Top with the cheese and oregano, and season with salt and pepper. Drizzle with the oil and bake for 15 minutes or until the tomatoes are tender.

Roasted Garlic Cauliflower Mash

....

Preparation time: **20 minutes** | Cooking time: **45 minutes**
Serves **4**

Cauliflower is a healthy replacement to use instead of mashed potatoes – and with creamy roasted garlic it really is delicious.

1 garlic bulb
2 tsp olive oil
1 large cauliflower, broken into small florets
4 tsp extra-virgin olive oil
75ml skimmed milk
2 tbsp freshly grated Parmesan cheese
1 tsp butter
1 tbsp low-salt vegetable bouillon powder
salt and freshly ground black pepper
snipped fresh chives, to garnish

1. Preheat the oven to 200°C/400°F/Gas 6. Peel away the outer papery layers of the garlic bulb skin, but leave the skin of each clove intact. Using a sharp knife, cut off about 5mm from the top of the cloves so that you can see the garlic inside the skin.

2. Put the bulb in a very small baking dish. Drizzle the olive oil over the garlic and use your fingers to coat the garlic cloves with the oil. Cover the dish with foil, then bake for 30 minutes or until the cloves are soft. The cloves will be very hot – leave to cool before handling.

3. Use a small knife to cut into the cloves and squeeze the soft garlic out with your fingers.

4. Put the cauliflower in a large pan and add water to a depth of about 2.5cm. Bring to the boil and then cook over medium-

high heat for 12–15 minutes until tender. Drain well in a colander.

5. Put the cauliflower into a food processor or blender and add 2 tsp of the extra-virgin olive oil, the garlic and all the remaining ingredients, then combine until thick and creamy. Serve drizzled with the remaining extra-virgin olive oil and garnished with chives.

Rice Pilaff

....

Preparation time: **10 minutes** | Cooking time: **50 minutes**
Serves **4**

Fragrant rice, piquant ginger, garlic and Indian spices – who could ask for more?

2 tbsp extra virgin olive oil
1 tsp mustard seeds
1 onion, chopped
1 large carrot, coarsely grated
2.5cm piece of fresh root ginger, peeled and grated
4 garlic cloves, crushed
2 dried bay leaves
½ tsp turmeric
1 tsp garam masala
1 tsp salt
400g brown basmati rice, rinsed
40g cashew nuts or chopped almonds
35g sultanas
1 litre vegetable stock
2 handfuls of fresh coriander, chopped

1. Heat the oil in a medium pan over medium-high heat, then add the mustard seeds. When they begin to pop, stir in the onion and carrot. Cook for 5 minutes or until the onion begins to soften, and then stir in the ginger, garlic, bay leaves, turmeric, garam masala and salt.

2. Stir well, then add the rice, nuts, sultanas and vegetable stock. Stir well, then cover, bring to the boil and simmer on low for 30–40 minutes until cooked completely. Stir in the fresh coriander and serve.

Apples with Creamy Peanut Dip

Preparation time: **10 minutes** | Serves **4**

Dip apples into this creamy peanut dip for a filling snack.

- 225g extra light soft cheese, softened
- 2 tbsp light muscovado sugar
- 1½ tsp vanilla extract or almond extract
- 2 tsp orange juice
- 2 tbsp coarsely chopped peanuts
- 4 apples, sliced

Put the softened cheese, muscovado sugar, vanilla extract and orange juice in a small bowl and mix until smooth. Stir in the chopped peanuts. Dip in the apples slices and enjoy!

Baked Cinnamon Apples

....

Preparation time: **5 minutes** | Cooking time: **30–40 minutes**
Serves **4**

When you're craving a sweet snack, reach for these delectably spiced baked apples.

4 cooking apples, such as Bramley
4 tbsp muscovado sugar
4 tsp butter
½ tsp ground cinnamon, or to taste
¼ tsp ground cloves, or to taste

Preheat the oven to 190°C/375°F/Gas 5. Core the apples and stand them upright in a 20cm square baking dish. Put 1 tbsp sugar in the centre of each apple, and add 1 tsp butter and a pinch of cinnamon and cloves (or more if you like a spicier taste). Pour 50ml water into the pan and bake for 30–40 minutes until the apples are soft.

Vanilla Poached Pears

....

Preparation time: **10 minutes** | Cooking time: **15–30 minutes**
Serves **4**

This traditional autumn favourite can be enjoyed almost all year round when pears are available. The pears are great served warm but they can also be chilled and eaten cold as a snack – what a treat!

4 Conference pears
zest of 1 lemon
juice of ½ lemon
2 tbsp maple syrup
1 cinnamon stick (optional)
1 tbsp sugar
1 tsp butter
1 tsp vanilla extract

1. Peel the pears and, using an apple corer, core them from the base end but leave the stems intact. Put the pears in a pan that is large enough to keep them upright and add the lemon zest and juice, the maple syrup and the cinnamon stick, if using. Cover with water. Bring to the boil, then reduce the heat and simmer over low heat for 15–30 minutes until the pears are tender when pierced with a knife.

2. Remove from the heat and allow the pears to completely cool in the poaching liquid. Remove the pears to serving plates and bring the poaching liquid to a fast boil. Stir in the sugar, butter and vanilla extract, and cook over a low heat until the sauce has reduced to a slightly thickened pouring consistency. Drizzle the sauce over and around the pears.

SAUCES, DIPS, DRESSINGS AND SPREADS

Basil Lime Sauce

....

Preparation time: **5 minutes** | Cooking time: **10 minutes**
Serves **4**

Basil and lime together create a lively taste sensation that promises to brighten simple rice or pasta dishes.

> 475ml dry white wine
> 1–2 garlic cloves, to taste, crushed
> 1 shallot, finely chopped
> 2 tsp sugar
> 2 tbsp lime juice
> 1 tbsp butter
> 1 large handful of fresh basil leaves, chopped

1. Heat a frying pan over medium-high heat and add the wine, garlic, shallot, sugar and lime juice. Bring to the boil, then immediately reduce the heat. Simmer for 8–10 minutes until the sauce reduces by half.

2. Turn off the heat and add the butter, then stir until melted. Leave to cool for 10 minutes, then stir in the basil leaves before serving.

Avocado-Corn Salsa

....

Preparation time: **10 minutes** | Serves **2**

This spicy salsa pairs well with baby carrots, courgette and cucumber slices.

½ avocado, stoned, peeled and diced
70g sweetcorn
1 plum or vine-ripened tomato, seeded and chopped
2 tsp chopped fresh coriander
lime juice, to taste
salt

Combine the avocado, sweetcorn, tomato and fresh coriander in a small bowl. Add lime juice and salt to taste.

Orange and Avocado Salsa

....

Preparation time: **15 minutes** | Serves **4**

Spoon this vibrant salsa over grilled chicken or salmon. Bursting with a bright citrus flavour, creamy avocado and the colourful taste of fresh coriander, it reminds you of summer, no matter what time of year it is.

4 large oranges
2 large pink grapefruits
½ red onion, finely chopped
2 tbsp chopped fresh coriander
1 tbsp chilli, seeded and finely chopped
2 tsp lime juice
1 avocado, stoned, peeled and diced
salt

1. Cut off the peel from the oranges and grapefruits using a small, sharp knife, then cut the juicy segments away from the white membranes. Cut the citrus segments into small pieces.

2. In a medium bowl, combine the fruit pieces, onion, fresh coriander, chilli, lime juice and avocado. Season with salt and serve.

Bean and Herb Dip

....

Preparation time: **5–7 minutes** | Serves **8**

This is a hearty dip for vegetables or rice cakes, or to use as a spread on wholemeal toast.

900g canned or fresh cooked cannellini beans
3 garlic cloves, crushed
3 tbsp lime or lemon juice
2 tbsp olive oil
2 tbsp chopped fresh basil
2 tbsp chopped fresh parsley
1 tbsp chopped fresh thyme, or ½ tsp dried thyme
salt and freshly ground black pepper

Drain and rinse the beans if using canned. Put all the ingredients in a food processor and purée until smooth and creamy.

Savoury Yogurt Dip

....

Preparation time: **5 minutes** | Serves **1**

This peppery dip will spice up any crudité tray.

  60g fat-free Greek yogurt
  ½ tsp lemon juice
  ¼ tsp lemon zest
  1 tbsp each chopped fresh thyme, dill, basil and coriander (or
     a few pinches of dried oregano, basil and thyme)
  salt and freshly ground black pepper

Put all the ingredients into a small food processor, then pulse
until smooth.

Low-fat Edamame Dip

....

Preparation time: **5 minutes** | Cooking time: **5 minutes**
Serves **8**

*Edamame provide the perfect base for this flavoursome hummus-like
dip to eat with fresh, crispy vegetables.*

  150g frozen edamame (soya beans)
  1 tbsp extra-virgin olive oil
  ½ tsp salt
  ½ tsp ground cumin
  2 garlic cloves, peeled
  1 handful of parsley leaves
  3 tbsp tahini
  3 tbsp fresh lemon juice

1. Cook the edamame according to the pack instructions, but do not add any salt. Drain.

2. Put the olive oil, salt, cumin and garlic in a food processor. Pulse a few times until coarsely chopped. Add the edamame, parsley, tahini, lemon juice and 3 tbsp water, then process for 1 minute or until smooth.

Red Kidney Bean Hummus Spread

....

Preparation time: **5 minutes** | Serves **8**

Pulses are a savoury treat, especially when blended with a little olive oil and tahini. Spread on a wholemeal tortilla and add beansprouts, tomatoes, lettuce, onions and any other vegetable you like. It's sure to be a hit!

400g can chickpeas, drained and rinsed
400g can red kidney beans, drained and rinsed
2 garlic cloves, crushed
1 tbsp olive oil
1 tbsp tahini
2 tbsp lemon juice, or to taste
2 tsp cumin

Put all the ingredients in a food processor and pulse for 2–3 minutes until very smooth. Add a little water if needed to thin to your preferred consistency.

Salmon Spread

....

Preparation time: **10 minutes** | Serves **12**

Use canned or leftover crumbled salmon for this tantalising spread. Use rice cakes or fresh veggies for dipping.

  2 x 213g cans pink salmon (without bones and skin)
  85g extra light soft cheese, softened
  115g fat-free Greek yogurt
  1–2 tsp creamed horseradish, to taste
  1 tsp lemon juice
  1 slice of mild onion, finely chopped

In a medium bowl, mix all the ingredients together and press into a 0.5-litre serving dish.

Chilli Lime Dressing

....

Preparation time: **5 minutes** | Serves **6–8**

This dressing will infuse a crisp salad with Asian-inspired flavours.

  3 tbsp soy sauce
  50ml lime juice
  2 tbsp muscovado sugar
  2 tsp Thai chilli sauce

Whisk all the ingredients together in a small bowl.

Honey Garlic Balsamic Vinaigrette

....

Preparation time: **5 minutes** | Serves **6–8**

Sweet and slightly tangy, this robust dressing tastes great with any salad.

   6 tbsp extra-virgin olive oil
   3 tbsp aged balsamic vinegar
   1 garlic clove, crushed
   ½ tsp honey
   2 tbsp water

Put all the ingredients in a small food processor and pulse until combined.

Lemon Caper Vinaigrette

....

Preparation time: **10 minutes** | Serves **4**

Salty capers and astringent lemon make perfect companions in a mix of heart-healthy olive and flaxseed oils.

   120ml extra-virgin olive oil
   50ml flaxseed oil
   50ml white balsamic or champagne vinegar
   4 tsp lemon juice
   4 tbsp capers, drained
   freshly ground black pepper

Combine all the ingredients thoroughly in a blender or salad dressing shaker to emulsify the oil and vinegar.

Sesame Miso Dressing

....

Preparation time: **5 minutes** | Serves **6–8**

Try sesame miso dressing on your favourite salad when you're in the mood for an Asian-inspired dish.

- 2 tbsp sesame seeds, plus extra to garnish
- 75ml rice wine vinegar
- 4 tbsp white miso
- 2 tbsp lemon juice
- 2 tsp grated ginger
- 1 tbsp sugar
- 1 tsp toasted sesame oil
- 3 tbsp mirin or cooking sake

In a small frying pan, toast the sesame seeds over high heat, shaking the pan constantly, for 2–3 minutes until the seeds begin to pop. Whisk all the ingredients together in a small bowl.

Sweet and Spicy Sesame Dressing

....

Preparation time: **5 minutes** | Serves **6–8**

Why decide between sweet or spicy? You can have both with this dressing.

- 2 tbsp toasted sesame oil
- 1 tbsp rice vinegar
- 1 tbsp balsamic vinegar
- 1 tsp hot chilli sauce
- 1 tsp agave nectar

Whisk all the ingredients together in a small bowl.

Thai Peanut Dressing

·······················

Preparation time: **5 minutes** | Serves **6–8**

If you're a fan of Thai food, you'll love this easy recipe for peanut dressing, a Thai staple.

- 250ml low-salt, fat-free chicken stock
- 2 tbsp smooth peanut butter, no added sugar
- 1 tbsp soy sauce
- 1 tsp lime zest
- 2 tbsp lime juice
- 2 tsp toasted sesame oil

Whisk all the ingredients together in a small bowl.

DESSERTS

Cherries with Ricotta and Toasted Almonds

....

Preparation time: **2–4 minutes** | Cooking time: **5–6 minutes**
Serves **2**

In just 5 minutes, you can be enjoying a dessert that will remind you of a cherry cheesecake.

> 115–150g cherries, stoned
> 2 tbsp low-fat ricotta cheese
> 1–2 tbsp toasted slivered almonds

1. Put the cherries in a small pan with 1 tbsp water then heat over medium heat for 5–6 minutes until they are warmed through.

2. Transfer to a small ovenproof bowl. Top the cherries with the ricotta, then scatter over the almonds. If you like, you can slide the dessert under a preheated grill for just a few seconds until the almonds are golden, but not for too long or they will burn.

Apple Cinnamon Brown Rice Pudding

....

Preparation time: **10 minutes** | Cooking time: **1 hour 10 minutes** | Serves **4–6**

Although this sinless dessert takes a bit of pot watching and time, it's well worth the effort.

200g brown rice
a pinch of salt
1 litre skimmed milk
1 tbsp agave nectar
3 tbsp maple syrup
1 tsp vanilla extract
2 tsp ground cinnamon
a pinch each of freshly grated nutmeg and ground cloves
130g raisins
1 large apple, peeled, cored and finely chopped

1. Combine 475ml water, the rice and salt in a large heavy-based pan. Bring to the boil over medium-high heat, stir once and cover with a tight-fitting lid. Reduce the heat to low and simmer for 40 minutes or until most of the water is absorbed. Remove the rice from the heat, transfer to a bowl and set aside.

2. In the same pan, add the milk, agave nectar, maple syrup, vanilla extract, cinnamon, nutmeg and cloves. Bring gently to the boil over medium heat, stirring frequently so that the milk doesn't burn, then reduce the heat to medium-low. Add the cooked rice, raisins and chopped apple, reduce the heat to low and simmer for 30 minutes or until the milk reduces and the rice is creamy. Stir frequently to prevent scorching.

3. Divide the pudding into 4–6 small bowls and serve warm or cold. If serving cold, cover with clingfilm to prevent the pudding from forming a skin on top while chilling.

Apple and Cranberry Crumble

....

Preparation time: **15 minutes** | Cooking time: **15 minutes**
Serves **9**

Healthy, fibre-packed wholemeal flour and oats makes this a satisfy-ing version of a old favourite with a twist.

oil spray
4 large cooking apples, peeled, halved and cut into thin slices
30g dried cranberries, naturally sweetened if available
1 tbsp plus 55g light muscovado sugar
3 tbsp plain wholemeal flour
2 tbsp rolled oats
2 tbsp butter

1. Preheat the oven to 230°C/450°F/Gas 8. Spray a 23cm square ovenproof dish with oil spray.

2. In a large pan, combine the apples, cranberries, 1 tbsp water and 1 tbsp muscovado sugar. Cook over medium-low heat for 5–6 minutes until the apples begin to soften. Stir occasionally to prevent sticking.

3. Meanwhile, put the flour, oats, butter and the remaining muscovado sugar in a small bowl, then combine with your fingers until crumbly. Set aside.

4. Put the hot apple mixture in the dish. Sprinkle the crumb mixture evenly over the top. Bake for 8–10 minutes until lightly browned and hot throughout.

Figgy Biscuits

....

Preparation time: **15 minutes** | Cooking time: **13 minutes**
Makes **24** (Serving size: **2** biscuits)

Remember fig rolls? These biscuits are an improvement on goodness, flavour and fibre. You can enjoy them without guilt.

115g butter
120g apple sauce from a jar, unsweetened
110g muscovado sugar
100g caster sugar
4 tbsp skimmed milk
1½ tsp vanilla extract
335g spelt or plain wholemeal flour
1 tsp bicarbonate of soda
zest of ½ orange
1 tsp each of ground cinnamon and ground ginger
75g rolled oats
40g chocolate chips
45g flaked almonds
50g dried figs, finely diced

1. Preheat the oven to 180°C/350°F/Gas 4. Line a baking sheet with baking parchment. Put the butter in a bowl and add the apple sauce, sugars, milk and vanilla extract. Combine together well.

2. Add the flour, bicarbonate of soda, orange zest and spices. Stir until fully mixed, then stir in the oats, chocolate chips, almonds and figs.

3. Scoop spoonfuls of dough onto the baking sheet and flatten using the back of a spoon. Bake for 13 minutes or until golden, then transfer to a cooling rack to cool completely.

Granola Plum Mini-muffin Pastries

....

Preparation time: **10 minutes** | Cooking time: **15–25 minutes**
Serves **12** (Serving size: **2** muffins)

Flaxseed, wholemeal flour and prunes add a hint of fibre to these delicious dessert muffins.

    oil spray
    130g stoned prunes, chopped
    120g plain wholemeal flour
    60g plain flour
    120g fat-free or low-fat granola
    55g muscovado sugar
    3 tsp baking powder
    1 tsp cinnamon
    ½ tsp ground ginger
    42g ground flaxseed
    120ml warm water
    4 tbsp molasses
    2 tsp honey
    2 tbsp olive oil
    2 tbsp unsweetened apple sauce from a jar
    250ml skimmed milk
    1 tsp vanilla extract

1. Preheat the oven to 200°C/400°F/Gas 6 and spray 12 mini-muffin cups with oil spray. Put the prunes in a bowl and add boiling water to just cover. In a large bowl, combine the flours, granola, sugar, baking powder and spices, then set aside.

2. In a small bowl, whisk together the flaxseed and warm water. Add the molasses, honey, oil, apple sauce, milk and vanilla extract. Set aside. Strain the prunes and stir into the flour mixture. Add the molasses mixture to the flour and stir until just incorporated.

3. Spoon the batter into the muffin cups until about two-thirds full. Bake for 10–15 minutes, then lower the heat to 180°C/350°F/Gas 4 and bake for a further 5–10 minutes until a skewer inserted into the centre of a muffin comes out clean.

Peachy Oat Crumble

....

Preparation time: **10 minutes** | Cooking time: **30 minutes**
Serves **8**

Make this lovely crumble when fresh and juicy peaches are in season. If you can get frozen peaches, you can also enjoy this delectable crumble at other times of the year.

oil spray
8 ripe peaches, peeled, stoned and sliced
juice from 1 lemon
⅓ tsp ground cinnamon
¼ tsp freshly grated nutmeg
55g plain wholemeal flour
55g muscovado sugar
2 tbsp butter
25g rolled oats

1. Preheat the oven to 190°C/375°F/Gas 5 and lightly coat a 23cm pie dish with oil spray.

2. Arrange the peach slices in the pie dish, then sprinkle with lemon juice, cinnamon and nutmeg.

3. Put the flour and muscovado sugar in a small bowl and whisk together. Using your fingers, rub the butter into the flour mixture, then add the oats and stir to mix evenly. Spoon the flour mixture evenly over the peaches. Bake for 30 minutes or until the peaches are soft and bubbly and the topping is browned.

Grilled Fruit with Balsamic Syrup

....

Preparation time: **10–15 minutes** | Cooking time: **3–5 minutes**
Serves **6**

Fruit is sweet – and it gets sweeter when it's HOT!

1 small pineapple, peeled, cored and cut into rings
2 large mangoes, peeled, stoned and cut into quarters
2 large peaches, stoned and cut into quarters
1 banana, halved lengthways
1 tbsp extra-virgin olive oil
2 tbsp muscovado sugar
120ml balsamic vinegar
oil spray
chopped mint or basil leaves, to decorate

1. Put the pineapple, mangoes, peaches and banana in a large bowl and mix well. Drizzle the olive oil over the fruit and stir or shake the bowl to coat each piece. Add the muscovado sugar and toss to coat evenly. Set aside.

2. Heat the balsamic vinegar in a small pan over low heat, then simmer until the liquid has reduced by half, stirring occasionally to prevent burning. Remove from the heat and set aside.

3. Preheat the grill to medium-high and spray the grill rack with oil spray. Put the fruit on the rack. Grill for 3–5 minutes until the fruit begins to brown. Remove the fruit from the grill and arrange on serving plates. Drizzle with the balsamic syrup and decorate with mint or basil.

Smart Brownies

....

Preparation time: **10 minutes** | Cooking time: **30 minutes**, plus cooling | Serves **12**

This as a smarter way to make brownies – they taste just as good as the traditional ones and are good for you too.

oil spray
350g carrots, roughly chopped
200g spinach
1 box brownie mix (I like Betty Crocker)
50ml extra-virgin olive oil
4 tbsp apple sauce from a jar, unsweetened
2 eggs

1. Preheat the oven to 180°C/350°F/Gas 4. Spray a 20cm square baking dish with oil spray. Cook the carrots in boiling water to cover for 10–15 minutes until tender. Drain. Meanwhile, put the spinach in a pan with only the water left on the leaves after washing. Cover and cook over medium-high heat, shaking the pan occasionally, until tender. Drain and chop, then set aside. Put the carrots into a small food processor and blend to a purée, then set aside.

2. Put the brownie mix in a medium mixing bowl and add the olive oil, apple sauce and eggs. Combine well, then stir in the carrot purée and the spinach. Pour the batter (it will be thick) into the baking dish and press into the corners. Bake for 30 minutes or until a skewer inserted into the centre comes out clean. Transfer to a wire rack to cool completely, then cut into squares.

Lemon Custard
with Fresh Blueberry Sauce

....

Preparation time: **15 minutes** | Cooking time: **1 hour 5 minutes**, plus **4 hours** chilling | Serves **4**

Soft (or silken) tofu lends smoothness and a silky texture to this custard. Blueberry sauce adds a sweet tang to balance the tartness of the lemon.

> oil spray
> 120ml silken tofu
> 350ml skimmed milk
> 3 eggs
> 2 tbsp light muscovado sugar
> 2 tbsp agave nectar
> 1 tsp lemon zest
> ½ tsp vanilla extract
> ½ tsp lemon extract
> 90g all-fruit blueberry or blackberry jam
> 2 tbsp lemon juice
> 115g fresh blueberries

1. Preheat the oven to 150°C/300°F/Gas 2 and spray four small ramekins with oil spray. Put the tofu and 120ml of the milk in a blender or food processor and combine until smooth.

2. Crack the eggs into a small bowl, then whisk them thoroughly. Add the muscovado sugar, agave nectar, lemon zest and the extracts. Whisk the egg mixture with the tofu mixture and remaining milk until well blended.

3. Pour the mixture into the ramekins and put them in a large roasting tin filled with hot water to come halfway up the sides of the ramekins. Bake for 50 minutes or until the custards

are set at the edge but slightly loose at the centre. Take the ramekins out of the tin and leave for 15 minutes to set. Cover with clingfilm and chill for at least 4 hours.

4. To make the blueberry sauce, put the jam and lemon juice in a small bowl and whisk until well blended. Gently stir in the blueberries to keep them intact. Top the custards with the blueberry sauce.

Grandma's Low-fat Chocolate Pudding

Preparation time: **10 minutes** | Cooking time: **15 minutes**
Serves **4**

Diana's grandma made this recipe when she was little and it has become a traditional after-dinner treat.

100g caster sugar
3 tbsp cornflour
3 tbsp unsweetened cocoa powder
550ml skimmed milk
1½ tsp vanilla extract

Put the sugar, cornflour and cocoa into a small pan over medium heat and mix well. Gradually blend in the milk and continue cooking, stirring constantly, until the mixture thickens. Cook for 3 minutes, then add the vanilla extract. Divide among 4 small dessert bowls and serve.

Grapes and Walnuts with Lemon Sauce

....

Preparation time: **20 minutes**, plus **1–2 hours** chilling | Serves **4**

Here's the magic bullet for satisfying your sweet tooth with the fat-fighting duo of fruit and nuts.

120g low-fat crème fraîche
2 tbsp icing sugar
1 tsp lemon zest
1 tsp lemon juice
⅛ tsp vanilla extract
140g red seedless grapes
140g green seedless grapes
3 tbsp chopped walnuts

1. In a small bowl, whisk together the crème fraîche, icing sugar, lemon zest, lemon juice and vanilla extract. Cover and chill for 1–2 hours.

2. Divide the grapes among 4 wine glasses or ramekins. Add 2 tbsp of the lemon topping to each dish and top with the chopped walnuts.

SPA BEVERAGES

Applelicious Tonic

....

Preparation time: **5 minutes** | Serves **1**

A refreshing alternative to plain water.

   25ml tart cherry juice
   75ml apple juice from a carton
   75ml orange juice (freshly squeezed or from a carton)
   75ml pineapple juice from a carton
   ice, enough to fill shaker

Combine the juices in a large shaker. Fill with ice and shake for several minutes until well chilled.

Fuzzy Peach Sparkler

....

Preparation time: **2 minutes** | Serves **1**

Enjoy this refreshing concoction at any time of day – morning, noon or night.

   50ml peach nectar
   175ml sparkling water (or diet tonic for a sweeter taste)
   ice, to serve

Pour the peach nectar into a large glass and add the sparkling water. Stir until blended, then serve over ice.

Iced White Tea

....

Preparation time: **5 minutes**, plus infusing and cooling | Serves **4**

White tea's subtle flavour has been called soft, smooth, sweet and sexy.

> 4 white tea bags (or 12 tsp loose white tea)
> 1.2 litres water
> 1 tbsp plus 2 tsp Truvia
> 4 fresh mint leaves, to decorate

1. Put the tea bags in a heatproof jug and pour in 1 litre boiling water. Leave to infuse for 3–5 minutes, then chill.

2. Meanwhile, pour 250ml water into a small pan and add the Truvia and mint leaves. Bring to the boil, remove from the heat and leave to infuse until cool. Sweeten the white tea with the mint syrup, to taste, and decorate with mint leaves.

Cool Cucumber Cooler

....

Preparation time: **10 minutes** | Cooking time: **3 minutes**
Serves **8**

Chilling, refreshing, light and bright – the cucumber and lime notes in this drink are suitable for lazy summer afternoons.

> 3½ tbsp Truvia
> 5 cucumbers, peeled and coarsely chopped
> 1 litre chilled water
> 4cm piece fresh root ginger, peeled and chopped
> juice of 3 limes
> 4 handfuls of ice cubes

1. Pour 120ml water into a small pan and add the Truvia. Bring to the boil, then simmer for 3 minutes or until all the Truvia has dissolved, to make a simple syrup. Pour into a heat-proof bowl to cool.

2. Put the cucumbers, 1 litre of water and the fresh ginger into a blender or food processor, and purée on high speed until smooth – you may need to do this in batches. Strain the cucumber mixture through muslin into a large jug and discard the solids. Stir in 4 tbsp of the syrup and the lime juice. Serve over ice.

Chilli Caipirinha

Preparation time: **5 minutes** | Cooking time: **3 minutes**
Serves **1**

Inspired by the national cocktail of Brazil, this 'mocktail' has a hit of spiciness.

1 lime
½ chilli, halved and seeded
50ml simple syrup (see Cool Cucumber Cooler step 1, above)
ice cubes
sparkling water

Squeeze the juice from the lime and put into a shaker, then add the chilli and simple syrup. Fill with ice and shake vigorously, then pour into a tall glass and top with sparkling water.

Pomegranate Nectar

....

Preparation time: **5 minutes** | Serves **1**

Pomegranate juice is full of healthy antioxidants and, even better, it tastes great.

    50ml pomegranate juice
    175ml mango nectar
    120ml sparkling water

Pour the pomegranate juice into a large glass and add the mango nectar and sparkling water. Stir until blended.

Pomegranate Splasher

....

Preparation time: **5 minutes** | Serves **1**

The splash of lime adds a twist to the pomegranate juice.

    50ml pure pomegranate juice
    250ml sparkling water
    1 tsp lime juice
    ice cubes, to serve

Pour the pomegranate juice into a large glass and add the sparkling water and lime juice. Stir until blended, and serve over ice.

Shirley Temple

....

Preparation time: **10 minutes** | Cooking time: **1 hour 5 minutes**, plus **30 minutes** cooling (for the syrup) | Serves **6**

Add pomegranate syrup to just about any beverage to create your favourite 'mocktail'.

  50ml pomegranate syrup (see below)
  250ml diet ginger ale
  1 maraschino cherry, to decorate

Pour the pomegranate syrup into a large glass and add the ginger ale. Stir until blended. Serve with a cherry.

POMEGRANATE SYRUP

  1 litre pomegranate juice
  3½ tbsp Truvia
  1 tbsp lemon juice

Pour the pomegranate juice into a small pan and add Truvia and lemon juice. Bring to the boil over medium heat, and cook, stirring frequently, until the Truvia has completely dissolved. Reduce the heat to medium-low and cook for 1 hour or until the mixture has reduced to about one-third, almost the consistency of syrup. Remove from the heat and cool for 30 minutes. Transfer to a glass jar and cool completely.

The syrup can be stored in the fridge for 3 months.

Virgin Mojito

....

Preparation time: **5 minutes** | Serves **1**

This mocktail is so tasty, you could serve it at a party!

½ lime, cut into small pieces
6 large mint leaves
¾ tsp Truvia
ice cubes
350g sparkling soda

Put the lime in a 350ml glass and add the mint and Truvia. Mash together to release the juice and flavours. Fill the glass with ice almost to the top and top up with soda. Stir lightly.

Sparkling Watermelon Sipper

....

Preparation time: **10 minutes**, plus **3 hours** chilling | Serves **8**

Make a hot summer's day cooler with refreshing watermelon – this time in a glass!

1.5kg watermelon, peeled and cut into chunks
juice of 2 limes
1 tbsp, plus 2 tsp Truvia
ice cubes, to serve
8 lime wedges, to serve (optional)

1. Put one-third of the watermelon into a blender and add 250ml water. Blend until smooth then pour into a large jug. Repeat with another third of the watermelon and then the final third.

2. Add the lime juice and Truvia to the watermelon mixture and stir until well blended. Chill for at least 3 hours until very cold. When ready to serve, pour into glasses filled with ice cubes and decorate with a lime wedge, if you like.

Spiced Ginger Lemon Spritzer

....

Preparation time: **5 minutes** | Cooking time: **1 hour** | Serves **6**

Ginger has long been used as a tummy tonic for easy digestion and to quell queasiness. Enjoy this drink as an after-dinner tonic.

10cm piece fresh root ginger, peeled
zest of 2 lemons
3–4 cinnamon sticks, to taste
½ tsp cloves
¼ tsp freshly grated nutmeg
⅔ cup, plus 3 tbsp Truvia
2 litres sparkling water (or diet tonic for a sweeter taste)
6 lemon slices, to decorate

1. Cut the ginger into 2.5cm pieces. Put it in a small pan and add the lemon zest, cinnamon sticks, cloves, nutmeg, Truvia and 250ml water. Bring to a quick boil, then reduce the heat and simmer for 30 minutes until reduced. Strain into a small jug and leave to cool.

2. For each drink, add 50ml of the syrup to a glass and top with sparkling water. Decorate with a slice of lemon.

CHAPTER NINE

······

Quickie Rev Up Moves and Routines

Are you ready to resculpt your body so that you can have long, lean muscles and a slimmer, sexier shape? In this chapter, you will see just how easy it can be to maintain muscle mass so that you can boost your metabolism and blast fat faster than ever. With the unique two-in-one Quickie Rev Up routine, all it takes is 21 minutes, just four times a week. A 3-minute Dynamic Warm Up primes your body from head to toe and then you alternate between 60-second Rev Up Blasts and 2 minutes of Strength Training Moves. How simple is that?

All you have to do is move through the routine quickly without taking any breaks. Be sure to start at the appropriate level to reduce the risk of injury and maximise results. The chart below shows the basic structure of what your workout will look like each time you complete it.

Quickie Rev Up structure

Dynamic Warm Up	3 minutes
Strength Training Move	2 minutes
Rev Up Blast	1 minute

Strength Training Move	2 minutes
Rev Up Blast	1 minute
Strength Training Move	2 minutes
Rev Up Blast	1 minute
Strength Training Move	2 minutes
Rev Up Blast	1 minute
Strength Training Move	2 minutes
Rev Up Blast	1 minute
Strength Training Move	2 minutes
Rev Up Blast	1 minute

Remember, you will have the option to adjust the difficulty of the moves based on your fitness level.

- **Make it easier** Start with the 'make it easier' versions of the Quickie Rev Up Foundation Moves for at least two weeks. When they feel too easy for you, try the basic versions.
- **Basic move** Progress to the basic options of the five Quickie Rev Up Foundation Moves for at least two weeks before advancing to the 'rev it up' options.
- **Rev it up** Move on to the 'rev it up' versions of the five Quickie Rev Up Foundation Moves for at least two weeks before progressing to the Quickie Rev Up Advanced Moves.

Check out the Fitness Assessment on page 126 to see what level you should begin at. But never feel pressured to advance to the next level before you're ready. This is not a race!

Important!
Check with your doctor before starting any exercise programme.

QUICKIE REV UP VOCAB LESSON

Athletic stance You don't have to be a professional athlete to assume an athletic stance. But mastering this simple posture while working out can boost your performance and help reduce the risk of injury. Here's how you do it: stand with your feet approximately hip-width apart and your knees slightly bent as you look straight ahead and keep your shoulders down, your chest out and your back straight.

Split stance Start in an athletic stance, then keeping your feet hip-width apart, step one foot about 45–60cm forward. Make sure your front foot is flat on the floor while your back one is resting on the ball of the foot.

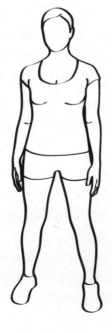

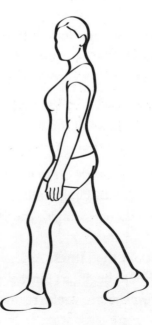

Athletic stance *Split stance*

Dynamic Warm Up moves

Do the following five Dynamic Warm Up moves in sequence for a total of three minutes.

EXERCISE **TWISTING HIGH KNEES**

What it exercises: front thighs, midsection

1. Start in an athletic stance with your arms bent in front of you.

2. Raise your left knee in front of you as you twist your upper body towards it, reaching the right elbow towards the knee.

3. Lower your left leg and return to the starting position.

4. Repeat on the right side, raising your right knee and twisting to the right. This completes one rep.

5. Keep alternating sides for 30 seconds.

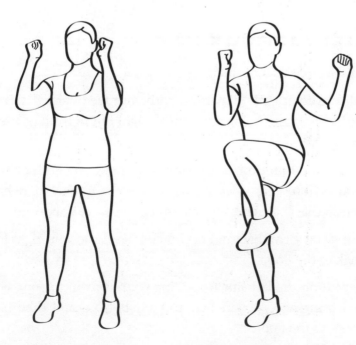

Twisting high knees (1)   *Twisting high knees (2)*

Make it easier Instead of touching your elbow to your knee, touch your hand to your knee.

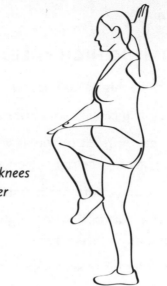

Twisting high knees – make it easier

EXERCISE **BOTTOM KICKS**

What it exercises: rear thighs

1. Start in an athletic stance but with your feet wider than hip-width apart and hold your arms straight out in front of you at shoulder level.

2. In one fluid motion, bend your arms and bring both of your elbows in to your sides and swing your right heel up behind you so that it touches – or comes close to – your bottom.

3. Bring your arms back out to shoulder level and your right foot back to the floor.

4. Repeat on the left side by pulling your arms in to your sides and bringing your left heel to your bottom and then back down to the floor.

5. Keep alternating from side to side for 30 seconds.

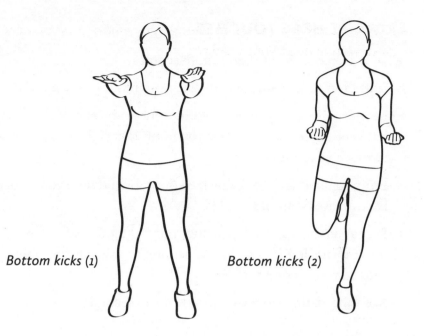

Bottom kicks (1)   *Bottom kicks (2)*

Make it easier Hold onto the back of a chair with two hands as you raise your feet.

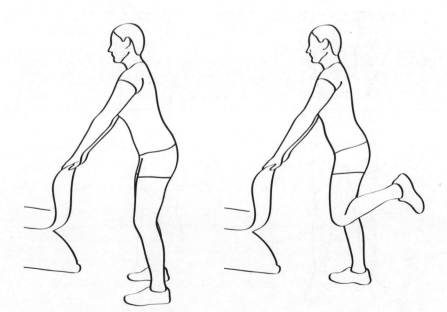

Bottom kicks – make it easier (1)   *Bottom kicks – make it easier (2)*

EXERCISE **HEEL TOUCHES**

What it exercises: front thighs, midsection

1. Start in an athletic stance with your arms raised over your head.

2. In one motion, lift your left foot in front of you and angle your left knee out to the side while you bring your right hand down to touch your left heel.

3. Bring your left foot back down to the floor and raise your arm back up over your head.

4. Repeat on the other side, raising your right foot and touching it with your left hand, then returning to the starting point. This completes one rep.

5. Keep alternating from side to side for 30 seconds.

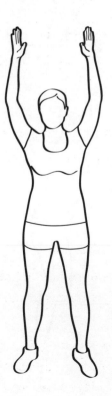

Heel touches (1)

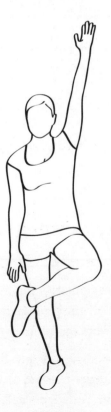

Heel touches (2)

Make it easier Start with your arms out to your sides at shoulder height, elbows bent, and touch the inside of your knee instead of your ankle.

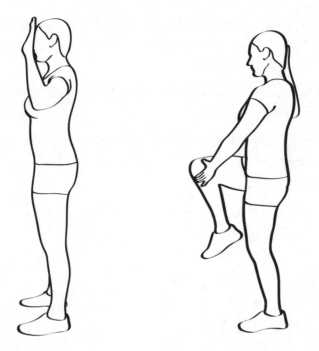

Heel touches – make it easier (1)   *Heel touches – make it easier* (2)

EXERCISE **LATERAL LEG SWINGS**

What it exercises: inner and outer thighs, midsection

1. Start by balancing on your left foot with your right foot hovering just off the floor in front of you and your arms out to the sides for balance.

2. Swing your right leg to the left as if you were using your foot to push a door closed as you swing your arms in the opposite direction. Your arms will help you balance. If you have trouble balancing, feel free to touch a table or the wall for support.

3. Without stopping, swing your leg back to the right as high as you can comfortably go, as your arms swing to the left. This completes one rep.

4. Swing your right leg from side to side for 30 seconds, then switch sides and swing your left leg from side to side for 30 seconds.

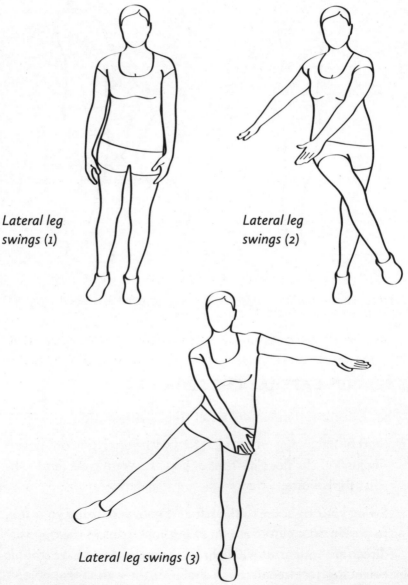

Lateral leg swings (1)

Lateral leg swings (2)

Lateral leg swings (3)

Make it easier Hold on to the back of a chair with one hand and put the other on your hip.

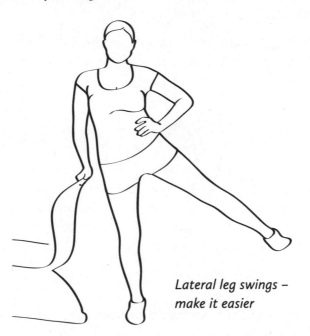

*Lateral leg swings –
make it easier*

EXERCISE **FRANKENSTEIN MARCH**

What it exercises: front thighs, rear thighs

1. Start in an athletic stance then raise your right leg straight out in front of you and try to touch your right toes with the fingertips of your left hand.

2. Bring your right leg and left hand down.

3. Raise your left leg straight out in front of you and reach for your left toes using your right hand.

4. Let your left leg and right hand return to the starting position. This completes one rep.

5. Keep alternating from side to side for 30 seconds.

See illustrations overleaf.

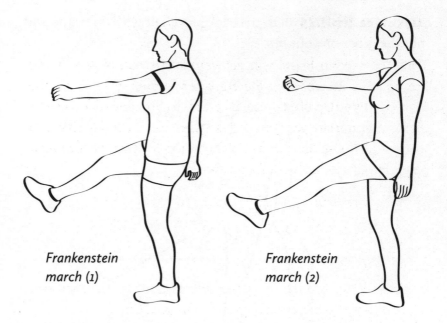

Frankenstein march (1)

Frankenstein march (2)

Make it easier Put your hands on your hips and raise your legs with your knees bent.

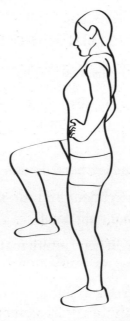

Frankenstein march – make it easier

Rev Up Blasts

These 60-second blasts will get your heart pumping and will fire up your metabolism. Here are ten simple ways to do the 60-second Rev Up Blasts. You're certain to find one that you love that is appropriate for your fitness level. On each day that you work out, choose one Rev Up Blast option for that day or mix it up with multiple options. It's up to you.

1. **Walk fast** Walk as fast as you can.

2. **Walk uphill** Walk uphill as fast as you can.

3. **Sprint** Run as if you were running away from someone scary.

4. **Walk/jog up stairs** Walk briskly or jog up stairs. When this feels comfortable, try taking two steps at a time.

5. **Jog on the spot** Bring your knees up high to your chest as you jog on the spot.

6. **Step up and down** Step up on a stair or step with one foot, then the other foot, then step down one foot at a time. Keep stepping up and down as quickly as possible.

7. **Repeaters** Step up on a stair or step with one foot, making sure that your standing leg is bent. Bring the knee of your other leg up to your chest then back down, lightly tapping your foot on the floor before raising your knee back up. Keep raising and lowering your knee for 30 seconds, then switch sides, stepping off the step and bringing your other foot onto the step and raising the opposite knee for the remaining 30 seconds.

8. **Jumping Jacks** You know the drill. However, if you aren't ready for jumping jacks, start in an athletic stance and instead of jumping, simply raise up onto your toes as you swing your arms overhead.

9. **Quick feet** This is similar to a drill commonly used in football training. Starting from an athletic stance with your feet wider

than hip-width apart, lean your upper body slightly forward and run on the spot as quickly as you can.

10. **Toe touch jumps** Starting from an athletic stance with your feet wider than hip-width apart, raise both arms up over your head. Crouch down and touch your toes, then jump as you rise back up and raise your arms back up over your head. Make sure your knees are slightly bent when you land, and immediately go back into your crouch.

WORKOUT TIP

Breathe easy!

Many people tend to hold their breath while working out, but this habit can cause lightheadedness, may cause you to strain your back and can make exercises seem even harder than they are. Remembering to breathe normally helps prevent injuries and eases you through challenging exercises.

Strength training moves

Regardless of your fitness level, it is best to master the five Quickie Rev Up Basic Foundation Moves before tackling the Quickie Rev Up Advanced Moves.

Quickie Rev Up Foundation Moves

EXERCISE **BRIDGE**

What it exercises: buttocks, rear thighs and the muscles that support the lower back

1. Lie on your back on the floor and bend your knees.

2. Tuck your pelvis under and lift your hips off the floor. Form a straight slope with your body from your shoulders to your knees.

3. Hold for 30 seconds, then relax for 10 seconds. Repeat twice more.

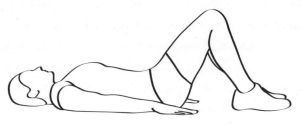

Bridge (1)

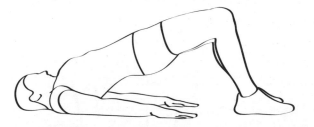

Bridge (2)

Make it easier Don't lift your hips off the floor. Just tuck in your pelvis so that you feel your back make contact with the floor.

Rev it up With your hips lifted, raise your right foot off the floor and straighten your right leg, keeping it parallel to your left leg. Hold for 15 seconds, then bring your right foot back down and straighten your left leg and hold for another 15 seconds. Bring your left foot back down and rest for 10 seconds before repeating the sequence.

EXERCISE **PLANK**

What it exercises: midsection, chest, front shoulders, back of the arms

1. Lie face down with toes tucked under and forearms on the floor.

2. Pull your belly up and in and raise your hips off the floor so that your body forms a straight line from your shoulders to your hips – a plank. Your elbows should be bent at a 90-degree angle directly under your shoulders. Keep your back straight – don't let your bottom pop up in the air or let your hips sag down towards the floor.

3. Squeeze in your midsection constantly, and hold this position. Don't forget to breathe.

4. Hold for 30 seconds, then relax for 10 seconds. Repeat twice more.

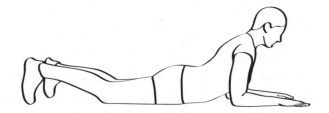

Plank (1)

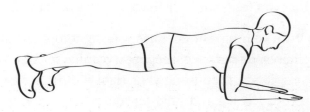

Plank (2)

Make it easier Drop your knees to touch the floor while maintaining your alignment.

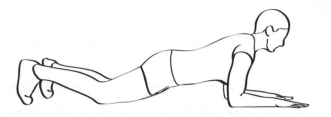

Plank – make it easier

Rev it up Straighten your arms into a full push-up position while maintaining your alignment.

QUICKIE REV UP VOCAB LESSON

Core vs midsection

What's the difference between your core and your midsection? Your midsection is what you typically think of as your abs – the muscles in your abdomen and on the sides of your waist. Your core also includes a group of muscles that support your back.

EXERCISE SQUAT

What it exercises: buttocks, front thighs, rear thighs, core

1. Start in an athletic stance and contract your midsection as you lower your bottom as if you were going to sit in a chair. Don't let your hips sink lower than your knees and don't let your knees jut further forward than your toes. Reach forward with your arms for balance.

2. Contract your buttocks and thighs to press back up to standing.

3. Do as many as you can in 30 seconds, then relax for 10 seconds. Repeat twice more.

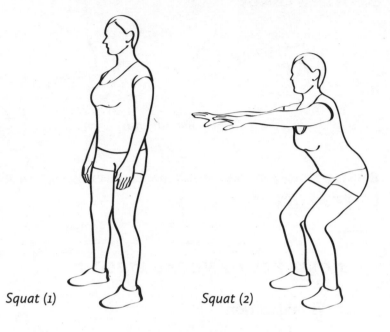

Squat (1)   *Squat (2)*

Make it easier Place a chair behind you and let your bottom touch the chair momentarily before coming back to standing.

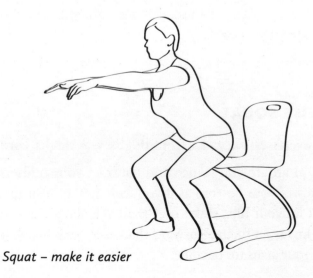

Squat – make it easier

Rev it up As you come back to standing, raise your arms overhead or add a jump.

EXERCISE **LUNGE**

What it exercises: calves, rear thighs, front thighs, inner and outer thighs, buttocks

1. Start in a split stance with your right foot in front.
2. Lower your hips until your left knee is almost touching the floor. Make sure your right knee is in line with your right toes, but not in front of them.
3. Engage the muscles in your legs to come back up to standing.
4. Do as many reps as you can in 30 seconds, then switch sides and repeat for 30 seconds. Repeat one more time on each side.

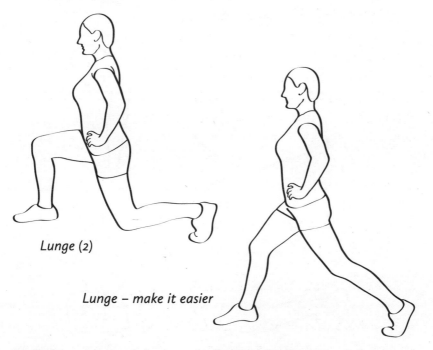

Lunge (2)

Lunge – make it easier

Make it easier Don't lower your hips as much.

Rev it up When you come back to standing, raise both arms overhead.

EXERCISE **PUSH-UP**

What it exercises: chest, front shoulders, rear arms, midsection

1. Start in a push-up position with the palms of your hands on the floor slightly wider than your shoulders and your knees touching the floor. Pull in your midsection and keep your body in a straight line from your knees to your head like in a plank. Don't let your bottom pop up in the air or sag down to the floor.

2. Bend your elbows as you lower yourself down towards the floor, keeping your body in that straight line.

3. Push back up to the start position, maintaining the same position with your body.

4. Do as many as you can in 30 seconds, then relax for 10 seconds. Repeat twice more.

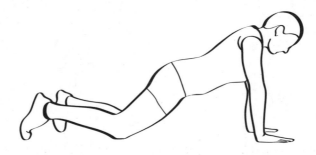

Push-up (1)

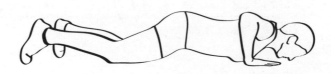

Push-up (2)

Make it easier Instead of lying face down, stand facing a wall and put the palms of your hands on the wall at shoulder level but slightly wider than your shoulders. Move your feet back about 30–60cm so that you are leaning at an angle. Push against the wall until your arms are fully extended, then return to the starting position.

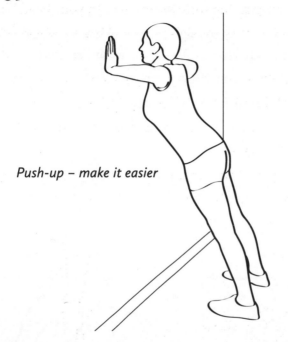

Push-up – make it easier

Rev it up Start with your knees lifted off the floor and your toes tucked under.

WORKOUT TIP

Bend it

To reduce the risk of injury, avoid locking out your knees and elbows while strength training. Maintain a slight bend to protect your joints.

Advanced Quickie Rev Up Moves

EXERCISE **WALL SIT**

What it exercises: front thighs, rear thighs, buttocks, calves

1. With your back flat against a wall, and your feet hip-width apart about 60cm away from the wall, slide down until your hips are at a 90-degree angle and your knees are directly over your ankles. Adjust your feet if necessary so that your knees are aligned with your ankles.

2. Hold the position for 30 seconds, then relax for 10 seconds. Repeat twice more.

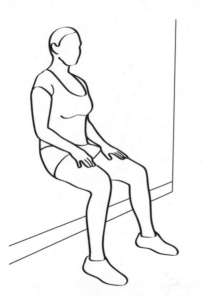

Wall sit (1)

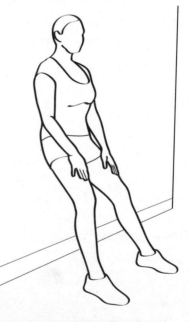

Wall sit – make it easier

Make it easier Don't slide down the wall quite as far.

Rev it up Hold the position for 50 seconds, then relax for 10 seconds. Repeat one more time.

EXERCISE **SIDE PLANK**

What it exercises: midsection, shoulders, rear arms, core

1. Lie on your left side with your left forearm on the floor and your elbow directly below your left shoulder. Keep your legs straight with your right leg stacked directly on top of your left leg.

2. Pull in your midsection as you lift your hips and knees off the floor to create a straight line with your body. Keep your head in line with your spine and don't let your hips pop up in the air or sag towards the floor.

3. Hold for 30 seconds, then return to the start position and switch to the other side. Repeat one more time on each side.

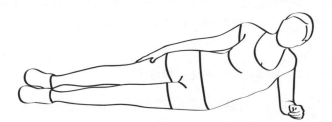

Side plank (1)

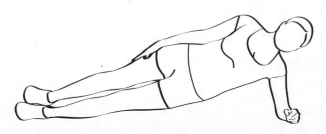

Side plank (2)

Make it easier Put your right knee on the floor in front of the left for stability.

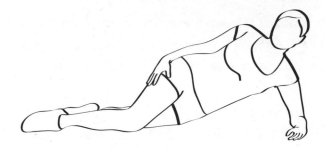

Side plank – make it easier

Rev it up With your hips lifted off the floor, raise your upper leg a few centimetres off your lower leg and raise the arm that isn't supporting you towards the ceiling to form a star.

EXERCISE **WALKING LUNGES**

What it exercises: calves, front thighs, rear thighs, inner and outer thighs, hips, buttocks

1. Start in an athletic stance.

2. Step forward with your left foot and lower your hips until your right knee is almost touching the floor. Make sure your left knee does not jut past your left toes.

3. In one fluid motion, engage the muscles in your legs and come back up to standing as you step forward with your right foot.

4. Step forward with your right foot and lower your hips until your left knee is almost touching the floor. Make sure your right knee does not jut past your right toes.

5. Keep alternating sides as you walk and lunge.

6. Do as many reps as you can in 30 seconds, then relax for 10 seconds. Repeat twice more.

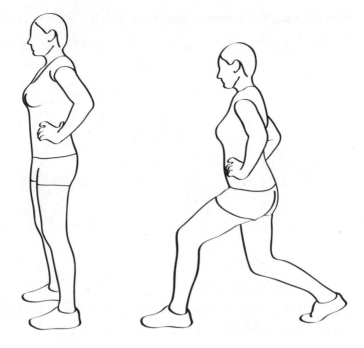

Walking lunges (1)   *Walking lunges (2)*

Make it easier Don't lower your hips as much.

Rev it up When you come back to standing, pull the knee of your back leg up to your chest and raise your opposite arm over your head.

EXERCISE **LUNGE AND TWIST**

What it exercises: calves, front thighs, rear thighs, inner and outer thighs, buttocks, midsection, core

1. Start in a split stance with your left foot forward, and bend your arms so that your hands are in line with your shoulders.

2. Lower your hips until your right knee comes close to the floor. At the same time, twist your upper body to the left.

3. Return to the start position.

4. Do as many reps as you can in 30 seconds, then switch sides and repeat for 30 seconds. Repeat one more time on each side.

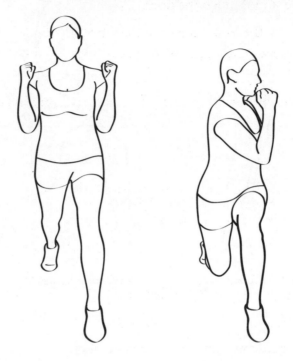

Lunge and twist (1)   *Lunge and twist (2)*

Make it easier Don't go as low when you lunge.

Rev it up When you rotate your upper body to the left, extend your right arm.

EXERCISE MOUNTAIN CLIMBERS

What it exercises: chest, front shoulders, rear arms, front thighs, rear thighs, buttocks, midsection

1. Start in a push-up position with your arms extended, your hands directly under your shoulders, and your toes tucked

under. Keep your body in a straight line, not allowing your bottom to pop up in the air or sag down to the floor.

2. Bring your right knee in towards your chest and let the ball of your right foot touch the floor.

3. Return to the start position then bring your left knee in towards your chest and let the ball of your left foot touch the floor.

4. Alternate from side to side for 30 seconds, then relax for 10 seconds. Repeat twice more.

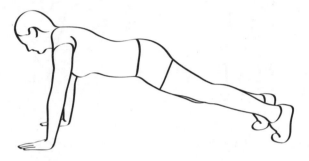

Mountain climbers (1)

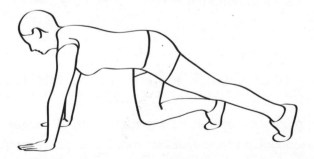

Mountain climbers (2)

Make it easier Start in an athletic stance. At the same time, raise your right arm straight over your head and lift your left knee. Return to the start then raise your left arm and right knee.

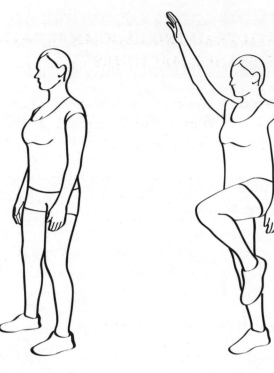

Mountain climbers –
make it easier (1)

Mountain climbers –
make it easier (2)

Rev it up Jump and switch feet in the air as you go from side to side.

Take Your Quickie Rev Up to the gym

If you prefer to work out at a gym, then by all means take your Quickie Rev Up to the nearest one. For added variety, you can work the same muscles using equipment you will find at most gyms. As with this programme's body-weight moves, you can adapt the exercises you do on machines to your fitness level. To make moves easier, use lighter weights or do fewer repetitions. To rev it up, use heavier weights or perform more repetitions.

STRENGTH TRAINING RECOMMENDATIONS FOR RESISTANCE MACHINES

Exercise selection: Perform 8–10 resistance-machine exercises that cumulatively engage all of the major muscle groups.

Exercise resistance: Use a resistance that enables you to complete at least 8 repetitions but not more than 12 repetitions.

Exercise progression: Increase the exercise resistance by approximately 5 per cent whenever you complete 12 or more repetitions.

Exercise sets: Perform one perfect set of each exercise.

Exercise speed: Use a controlled movement speed of approximately 6 seconds per repetition, with 3 seconds for each lifting action and 3 seconds for each lowering action.

Exercise range: Use a complete movement range for each repetition, but never push yourself into painful positions.

Exercise breathing: Exhale during lifting actions and inhale during lowering actions; never hold your breath.

Here is a quick look at the gym equipment that is best to use for this workout. If you aren't familiar with these machines, ask a personal trainer or a gym employee for assistance in using them.

- Leg extension machine (what it exercises: front thighs)
- Leg curl machine (what it exercises: rear thighs)
- Leg press machine (what it exercises: front thighs, rear thighs, buttocks)
- Chest press machine (what it exercises: chest, front shoulders, rear arms)
- Pull down machine (what it exercises: upper back, front arms, forearms)
- Shoulder press machine (what it exercises: shoulders, rear arms)
- Mid-row machine (what it exercises: upper back, front arms, forearms)
- Abdominal machine (what it exercises: midsection)
- Low back machine (what it exercises: core)
- Rotary torso machine (what it exercises: midsection)

Keep it Revved Up

After just two weeks of doing the Quickie Rev Up, you will start to feel stronger, more energised, and more toned. You will be losing pounds without losing the lean muscle mass that gives your body definition. When you see results so quickly, it keeps you motivated, which makes it so much easier to stick with the routine. And when you regularly devote 21 minutes four times a week to the Quickie Rev Up, it keeps fat burning and weight loss revved up too.

The following charts illustrate two 2-Week Quickie Rev Up plans, one for basic moves and one for advanced moves.

2-Week Quickie Rev Up plan – basic moves

WEEK 1

DAY 1	DAY 2	DAY 3	DAY 4	DAY 5	DAY 6	DAY 7
1-Day Power Up	6-Day Fuel Up					
Rest day	**Dynamic warm-up**	Rest day	**Dynamic warm-up**	Rest day	**Dynamic warm-up**	**Dynamic warm-up**
	Bridge		Push-up		Lunge	Plank
	Walk fast		Jog on the spot		Walk fast	Jog on the spot
	Plank		Squat		Bridge	Push-up
	Walk fast		Jog on the spot		Walk fast	Jog on the spot
	Squat		Plank		Squat	Plank
	Walk fast		Jog on the spot		Walk fast	Jog on the spot
	Push-up		Lunge		Lunge	Push-up
	Walk fast		Jog on the spot		Walk fast	Jog on the spot
	Lunge		Push-up		Bridge	Plank
	Walk fast		Jog on the spot		Walk fast	Jog on the spot
	Plank		Squat		Squat	Push-up
	Walk fast		Jog on the spot		Walk fast	Jog on the spot

continued

WEEK 2

DAY 1	DAY 2	DAY 3	DAY 4	DAY 5	DAY 6	DAY 7
1-Day Power Up	6-Day Fuel Up					
	Dynamic warm-up		Dynamic warm-up		Dynamic warm-up	Dynamic warm-up
	Squat		Push-up		Lunge	Push-up
	Step up & down		Repeaters		Step up & down	Repeaters
	Lunge	Rest day	Bridge		Squat	Plank
Rest day	Step up & down		Repeaters		Step up & down	Repeaters
	Plank		Plank	Rest day	Bridge	Plank
	Step up & down		Repeaters		Step up & down	Repeaters
	Squat		Lunge		Lunge	Push-up
	Step up & down		Repeaters		Step up & down	Repeaters
	Lunge		Push-up		Squat	Plank
	Step up & down		Repeaters		Step up & down	Repeaters
	Plank		Squat		Bridge	Plank
	Step up & down		Repeaters		Step up & down	Repeaters

2-Week Quickie Rev Up plan – advanced moves

WEEK 1

DAY 1	DAY 2	DAY 3	DAY 4	DAY 5	DAY 6	DAY 7
1-Day Power Up	6-Day Fuel Up					
Rest day	Dynamic warm-up	Rest day	Dynamic warm-up	Rest day	Dynamic warm-up	Dynamic warm-up
	Walking lunges		Mountain climbers		Squat	Mountain climbers
	Quick feet		Jumping jacks		Sprint	Walk uphill
	Side plank		Lunge		Lunge & twist	Side plank
	Quick feet		Jumping jacks		Sprint	Walk uphill
	Squat		Side plank		Wall sit	Push-up
	Quick feet		Jumping jacks		Sprint	Walk uphill
	Mountain climbers		Lunge & twist		Lunge	Plank
	Quick feet		Jumping jacks		Sprint	Walk uphill
	Wall sit		Plank		Squat	Side plank
	Quick feet		Jumping jacks		Sprint	Walk uphill
	Push-up		Squat		Walking lunges	Push-up
	Quick feet		Jumping jacks		Sprint	Walk uphill

continued

2-Week Quickie Rev Up plan – advanced moves (continued)

WEEK 2

DAY 1	DAY 2	DAY 3	DAY 4	DAY 5	DAY 6	DAY 7
1-Day Power Up	6-Day Fuel Up					
Rest day	**Dynamic warm-up**	Rest day	**Dynamic warm-up**	Rest day	**Dynamic warm-up**	**Dynamic warm-up**
	Mountain climbers		Walking lunges		Squat	Mountain climbers
	Jog upstairs		Toe touch jumps		Repeaters	Sprint
	Walking lunges		Plank		Lunge & twist	Side plank
	Quick feet		Jog on the spot		Jumping jacks	Quick feet
	Push-up		Squat		Wall sit	Push-up
	Jog upstairs		Toe touch jumps		Step up & down	Jog upstairs
	Side plank		Side plank		Walking lunges	Plank
	Quick feet		Jog on the spot		Repeaters	Sprint
	Lunge & twist		Wall sit		Squat	Mountain climbers
	Jog upstairs		Toe touch jumps		Jumping jacks	Quick feet
	Mountain climbers		Push-up		Lunge	Plank
	Quick feet		Jog on the spot		Step up & down	Push-up

PART 4

The Overnight Diet for Life!

....

CHAPTER TEN

The Overnight Diet Eating-out Guide

Life is full of happy, exciting occasions, and the vast majority of them centre around – you guessed it – food. Going out to dinner with friends, sharing holiday meals, meeting clients for lunch, attending weddings and birthday parties, seeing a film, and even going to a sports event are all occasions where food plays a supporting, if not a starring, role. You can learn to enjoy yourself at all of these types of events without shifting fat burning into reverse. With the simple guidelines in this chapter, you will keep the weight coming off while living your life to the fullest. And after all, isn't that what this is all about?

Eating out on the 1-Day Power Up

So what happens when your 1-Day Power Up falls on a day when you have to be out of town on a business trip? Or you're visiting your ailing Grandma who has never even heard of protein powder? Or you'll be spending a good portion of the day at the airport? Don't worry. Sticking with your 1-Day Power Up when you're travelling is easier than you think. It just takes a bit of planning, preparation and knowledge.

One of the best things you can do to keep from being caught unprepared is to carry single-serving bags of protein powder and a fibre supplement (if you're using Physicians Protein Mix you won't need a separate fibre supplement because it's already included in the mix and packaged for a single serving), or keep a stash of your favourite flavours of the Physicians Protein Smoothie handy. You just need enough to get you through one day, so they won't take up much room in your handbag, briefcase or suitcase. And they're light, so you won't be in danger of getting charged any excess baggage fees.

That way, when you get to Grandma's house, you can toss the protein powder into a blender with whatever fruit she has in the house and add a little bit of milk, or even just water, for a make-do smoothie. Or if you're using the Physicians Protein Smoothie, you just pick the flavour you want, add water and shake – no blender necessary. It may not be as inventive as the smoothies you can make at home, but it will do at a pinch to keep your metabolism fired up so you will lose weight overnight.

Tales of the Measuring Tape

'I went to visit my in-laws over the holidays so I took some protein powder with me for my 1-Day Power Up. They had frozen fruit in their freezer and skimmed milk in the fridge, so I just popped it all in their blender and *voilà*! It couldn't have been easier.' Josh, 37, lost 1 stone 12 pounds (11.8kg) and is down from a size 38 to size 34 trousers

What if you're nowhere near a blender and don't have your Physicians Protein Smoothie? Rest assured that smoothies have become so popular that you can probably find a smoothie wherever you are visiting. Many airports boast smoothie shops.

And fun, fruity concoctions are also popping up on menus at fast-food chains and coffee shops as well as in supermarket aisles.

All smoothies are not created equal, however. The recipes here and the Mix 'n' Match Smoothie Chart (page 346) have been carefully crafted – much work went into perfecting the combinations for maximum effect. It's unlikely, for example, that the owners of your local smoothie outlet have earned a medical degree, helped thousands of people lose weight, consulted with a registered dietician, know how lean muscle affects weight loss, understand how protein is the building block for muscle and are aware of the dangers of Shrinking Muscle Syndrome, or have analysed the latest research on satiety.

Some of their smoothies will be fat-filled calorie hogs with virtually no protein or fibre. So they will pack on the pounds and still make you feel hungry sooner rather than later. Even the 'Slim-Down Smoothie' that sounds so healthy might actually contribute to Shrinking Muscle Syndrome and those abundant curves on your hips. So how can you decipher the menu so that you know what to order?

Fortunately, most smoothie shops *do* have a few healthy options. You just have to be smart about how you order. In general, if you're looking for something that's going to prime your body for fat burning, keep it simple. The fewer the ingredients, the better. If you don't see anything on the menu that looks like it would earn 1-Day Power Up approval, don't be afraid to order off the menu. If you order a smoothie made with only the following ingredients, you should be in good shape – literally:

- Whey or soya protein: 24–28g of protein

- Fibre – at least 5g

- Skimmed milk, soya milk, water or ice

- Fresh or frozen fruit that isn't soaked in syrup

- Fat-free yogurt

With some of them, you'll still need to add a protein boost (to reach 24–28g protein) or a fibre boost (to get at least 5g fibre) to make it worthy of the 1-Day Power Up, so be sure you have your bags of protein and fibre on you at all times. Remember, shop-bought smoothies are for emergencies only. Don't make them a habit.

Tales of the Measuring Tape

'I used to order this smoothie that I thought was going to help me lose weight, but after I learned what to look for in a smoothie, I realised that the one I was drinking didn't have any protein and virtually no fibre. It was basically calories and sugar. No wonder I always felt so hungry right after I drank it. Now when I'm travelling, I know which smoothies to order and when I need to add a protein boost. And I can go for hours afterwards without my stomach growling.' Nikki, 24, lost 1 stone 2 pounds (7.2kg)

Eating out on the 6-Day Fuel Up

So you've cleaned all the junk food out of your cupboards and filled your kitchen with good-for-you fruits, vegetables, lean carbs, lean protein and healthy fats. You're eating a delicious, protein-packed, high-fibre lunch that keeps you satisfied all afternoon – no more vending machine calling your name at three o'clock. You're whipping up 15-minute and no-cook recipes at home and loving them and, even better, your jeans are feeling looser and your arms don't jiggle the way they used to. Way to go!

Now your colleagues have just invited you out to lunch to celebrate your office mate's birthday. What do you do? You know that many restaurants use cooking techniques and ingredients that are loaded with saturated fats, refined carbohydrates, sugar and salt, and that the portion sizes are often too large. All of these can be a recipe for weight gain, bloating and fat production. Should you just say no thanks and hide in your office while you eat the food you brought from home? There's no need to panic or shrink like a wallflower. Take a deep breath, arm yourself with the following tips and have a great time!

These simple strategies worked for Angela, who was almost 3½ stone (22.7kg) overweight when she visited the Nutrition and Weight Management Center at Boston Medical Center. She had tried to lose weight, but whenever she and her friends went out to eat, it turned into a free for all. She would always tell herself she wasn't going to overeat, but as soon as the waiter put the basket of bread on the table, she would dig in and her resolve would quickly evaporate. Then when she opened the menu, her eyes would dart quickly from one diet disaster to the next: cheese-burger with French fries, pasta with a creamy sauce, chicken pie. Sometimes she would give in and order the calorie bomb.

At other times she would choose something that she thought sounded healthy but it then turned out to be full of fat and cal-ories; for example, once she ordered a salad with peaches and grilled chicken. She thought to herself, 'It's peaches with grilled chicken – it must be healthy.' Wrong! Yes, it did have ample amounts of protein and fibre, but it was very high in calories and saturated fat. The list of ingredients offered clues that could have tipped her off to the big calorie count:

- Caramelised peaches – 'caramelised' means it's made with gobs of butter and sugar

- Dried cranberries – dried fruits like cranberries are often coated with lots of sugar

- Caramelised pecan nuts – more butter and sugar

- Feta cheese – probably full-fat

- Crispy breaded chicken – 'crispy' is a code word for 'fried' and foods are typically breaded with some form of refined flour

- Blue cheese dressing – one of the fattiest, highest-calorie dressings

On that particular day, Angela also downed two fizzy soft drinks and decided that since she had only had a salad, she would split a dessert with her friends. Even divided by the three of them, the dessert was still more than 450 calories apiece. Angela left the restaurant that day feeling bloated. By that evening, she realised she had already destroyed her diet so she ordered a pizza for dinner and had a huge helping of Häagen Dazs Dulce de Leche ice cream for dessert.

Angela needed some tips to help her make better choices when eating out. Here's what she learned.

Order off the menu

Most restaurants these days are very accommodating and will eagerly make substitutions. In fact, you don't even have to bother looking at the menu. You could just ask for the following:

- Grilled chicken breast or grilled, baked or poached fish – plain, without any butter or sauce
- Steamed vegetables
- Quinoa, brown rice or wholewheat pasta

Many restaurants will accommodate you. If a restaurant doesn't have any brown rice, quinoa or wholewheat pasta, you can always double up or even triple up on the vegetables. They may charge a little bit extra when you do this, but isn't it worth it to keep the fat coming off and to boost your health while you're at it?

Know before you go

Thanks to the Internet, it's easier than ever to check the menu – and in some cases the nutritional info – at restaurants before you sit down to peruse the menu. Whenever possible, choose your main course before you get to the restaurant. And then don't even open your menu at the table. Tune out when the waiter tells you about their 'amazing' specials and order first so that you aren't tempted by anyone else's order. Stick to the smart choice.

Decode the menu

Decrypting a menu is similar to translating a foreign language. Those ingenious restaurant marketing gurus slip in words that make some foods sound healthy when they really aren't. And sometimes the same culinary term might indicate a dish that gets the green light or one that you should skip; for example, baked fish gets a thumbs up but baked cookies don't. A pear salad can be a good choice, but a pear or apple crumble isn't. Clearly, it can get a bit confusing.

Knowing how to translate those culinary clichés will help you get an A+ in healthy ordering. You may want to keep the following lists with you as a sort of cheat sheet when dining out so that you can translate those menus and stay on track. The terms in the Green Light list are the ones that are likely to help you keep the weight coming off. The Yellow Light list is a little trickier because the terms may denote a healthy option in some cases but not in others. Read the descriptions of these terms for clarification. The Red Light list contains terms that typically indicate menu choices that slow your fat-burning engines and are more likely to pad your hips and thighs.

Green Light

Boiled
Grilled
Poached
Steamed
Whole grain

Yellow Light

Baked	Multi-grain
Crisp/crispy	Organic
Crunchy	Roasted
Fat-free	Sautéed
Fresh	Seasoned
Garnish	Spiced/spicy
Chargrilled	Stir-fried
Light/lite	Vegetarian
Marinated	Vinaigrette

Red Light

Au gratin	Creamy/creamed/cream sauce
Basted	Crumb coated/crumble
Battered	Crust/crusted
Breaded	Dip/dipping sauce
Buttered/butter sauce	Fried/deep-fried/pan-fried/flash-fried
Candied	Glazed
Caramelised	Herb crusted
Cheesy	Melted
Coated	Stuffed
Country-style	Tempura

Yellow light terms decoded

Baked: baked poultry and fish are great, but baked biscuits, cookies and muffins aren't.

Chargrilled: this means being cooked over intense heat. The cooking method is fine, as long as it isn't grilled in butter, but it depends on what is being grilled – a half-pound burger or a few prawns?

Crisp/crispy: crisp lettuce is good, but crispy coated chicken breast and crispy onion rings aren't.

Crunchy: crunchy vegetables get a thumbs up, but crunchy tortilla chips or croutons in your salad don't.

Fat-free: don't be fooled by the fat-free tag – just because it's fat-free doesn't mean you can order two or three. Many fat-free products have a higher sugar content.

Fresh: fresh tomatoes and other vegetables are great, but freshly baked pastries and fresh cheese may not help you reach your goal weight.

Garnish: if it's garnished with a parsley sprig, OK. If it's garnished with soured cream, garlic mayo or some other fattening sauce, say no thanks.

Chargrilled: this means being cooked over intense heat. The cooking method is fine, as long as it isn't grilled in butter, but it depends on what is being grilled – a half-pound burger or a few prawns?

Light/lite: light variations of meals may have fewer calories but may have also been stripped of fibre and protein.

Marinated: find out what it's marinated in – a sugary glaze (no thanks!) or red wine vinegar (OK). As a rule, look for marinades that are low in fat and low in sugar.

Multi-grain: multi-grain is not whole grain; skip it.

Organic: how can something organic be bad for your diet? When it's fried, breaded or smothered in a cream sauce.

Roasted: it may be roasted in a lot of oil so beware – ask if in doubt.

Sautéed: sautéed means that something is fried quickly. Ask for it to be sautéed in a small amount of oil or cooking spray.

Seasoned: being seasoned with herbs is ideal, but watch out if butter or oil is thrown into the mix.

Spiced/spicy: spices are a wonderful way to add flavour or a little kick. It's too bad restaurants also often add butter, fat or cream to these spices. Ask how it's prepared.

Stir-fried: this basically means fried quickly. Ask for it to be stir-fried in a small amount of oil or use cooking spray instead.

Vegetarian: just because something is meatless doesn't necessarily make it healthy. Vegetarian lasagna can be a cheesy mess that will slow down your metabolism, so be aware.

Vinaigrette: many places smother salads with too much dressing. Stick with vinaigrette and ask for it on the side.

Dining out

Not every restaurant prepares meals the same way, but there are some general guidelines you can follow at your favourite restaurant.

Chinese

Consider: appetisers with lettuce wraps; steamed dumplings; Sichuan dishes with sauces made from chicken stock, such as garlic sauce; whole steamed fish for sharing; steamed meats and vegetables.

Pass on: fried rice; fried wontons and spring rolls; moo shu pork; sweet-and-sour dishes; duck; nut dishes.

French

Consider: broth-based stews such as bouillabaisse; coq au vin; salade Niçoise.

Pass on: au gratin dishes, which are made with cheese, butter and sometimes cream; hollandaise or Béarnaise sauces; dessert pastries; quiches; pâté.

Greek

Consider: fish baked with garlic and tomato-based plaki sauce; shish kebab or any grilled lamb dish.

Pass on: avgolemono; baklava; moussaka; falafel; kibbeh.

Italian

Consider: Florentine dishes, usually chicken or veal dressed with spinach; pastas with tomato-based sauces; primavera pasta; clam sauce; mussels; polenta; pizza (one thin slice with oil blotted and topped with vegetables).

Pass on: sauces made with cream; pasta carbonara; pizza topped with sausage, pepperoni or other meats; pesto sauce.

Japanese

Consider: miso soup; sukiyaki; fish and vegetable sushi and sashimi; teriyaki (chicken, fish and beef).

Pass on: anything 'crispy'; fried meat; tempura.

Mexican

Consider: chicken enchiladas or burritos without cheese; salsas served with baked tortilla chips; ceviche; soft tacos; veracruz dishes, which are made from tomatoes, onions and chillies.

Pass on: anything made with soured cream and cheese; fried tortilla chips and taco shells; refried beans; chorizo.

Middle Eastern

Consider: anything made with couscous or tabbouleh; lavash; lentil dishes; Moroccan stew; baba ghanoush and hummus spreads.

Pass on: dips floating in oil; falafel; stuffed vine leaves, which usually come bathed in oil.

Thai

Consider: chicken satay (dip into the peanut sauce sparingly); hot and spicy soups; noodle bowls; steamed or grilled fish.

Pass on: coconut curries; pad thai.

Pay attention to portions

Once the preserve of the US, extra-large portions are now becoming more common in other countries. Some restaurants serve massive plates piled high with food and if your mum taught you to 'clean your plate', you probably think you're supposed to eat everything you are served. It's time for you to take control of the portions you eat. Some restaurants offer half portions, and even if you don't see it listed on the menu, ask if you can get a half portion if you're eating somewhere where portions are generally large. You can also split a main course with your dining partner or ask the waiter to put half of your meal in a takeaway container before bringing it to your table. To avoid ending up with a jumbo meal, avoid ordering menu items that use the following terms.

- **Combo** This usually indicates two meals in one, like steak and seafood.

- **Generous** 'Generous' portions will generate more fat cells.

- **Monster** Anything that's 'monster' sized will increase your size.

- **Value** Is it really a value meal if it makes you gain weight and harms your health?

On her next appointment to see me, Angela shared her latest restaurant experience. Once again, her friends had asked her to go out for lunch. This time, she jumped online to look at the restaurant's menu first. Based on the nutritional info, she decided on a roasted vegetable salad with grilled chicken – a half order, which most restaurants offer at lunch. You can typically order a lunch-sized portion at dinner, too. You just need to ask.

When they got to the restaurant, Angela asked the waiter to take the bread away from the table after her friends had taken their share from the bread basket. She ordered first so that she wouldn't be influenced by what her friends were ordering. She asked for fat-free vinaigrette on the side and only used about half of it. She stuck to water with her meal and when her friends mentioned dessert, Angela opted for a decaf iced cappuccino that was under 100 calories. Altogether, she shaved off almost 2,000 calories from her lunchtime meal. She left feeling pleasantly full and, best of all, good about her decisions. Later that night, she ate reasonably and woke up 1 pound (450g) lighter the next day.

What Angela realised is that with a few small tweaks, she could go out with her friends and still eat a healthy meal that tasted great and would help her to lose weight. You can too if you follow the guidelines in this chapter.

The festive season

Happy Christmas! Did you know that your friends, family, colleagues and employers are all chipping in to get you something? Do you want to know what it is? A spare tyre. Yes, all those well-meaning folks with their holiday meals, parties, cocktails and treats conspire to slow your metabolism to a screeching halt and cause your fat cells to start expanding like party balloons. The Overnight Diet is designed to help you combat typical over-Christmas weight gain. The 6-Day Fuel Up keeps hunger at bay and makes you less likely to experience intense cravings for fattening festive fare. And even if you overindulge at an event, the 1-Day Power Up can help put you back on track. Here are some sure-fire strategies to help you muscle through the festive season so that you can keep the weight coming off.

Eat before you go Have a healthy, high-protein, high-fibre snack or a small meal before that party or celebration meal. The protein and fibre will ensure that you won't be starving and tempted to grab every appetiser that comes your way. Don't have time for a meal with protein and fibre? Eat an apple on your way to the party. It can curb your appetite.

GET THE LOWDOWN ON THE SCIENCE

An apple on the way saves the day

Eating an apple 15 minutes before a meal reduces intake at that meal by 15 per cent, according to a study in *Appetite* from researchers at Penn State. This trial, which involved 30 men and 28 women, also showed that eating a whole apple caused a greater reduction in subsequent intake than having apple purée or apple juice with added fibre.

Go for the 6-Day Fuel Up-friendly foods first As soon as you arrive, search for any raw vegetables or fruit, lean protein like prawns or whole-grain crackers and take a small plate of them. Noshing on these foods will keep your mouth occupied and increase satiety so you are less likely to overindulge on the fattier fare.

Scout out the buffet, then choose With buffet-style meals, don't load up your plate as you go through the line. Scan all the offerings first, then take only the few things that you really love.

Don't park yourself next to the buffet Take the advice of Brian Wansink, a Cornell University professor and author of *Mindless Eating*, and sit as far away from the buffet as you can while you eat.

BYOD (bring your own dish), if it's OK with your hosts. Chicken and veggie skewers or a spinach salad with turkey breast is a good option that can look festive, plus you can make an entire meal out of them.

Get back on track So you overdid it at the office shindig. Don't beat yourself up about it. Just get back to the 1-Day Power Up or 6-Day Fuel Up depending on the day of the week.

Holidays

Just because you're going on holiday doesn't mean you have to take a holiday from your healthy eating habits. Whether you're hitting the slopes, sinking your toes in the sand, or hopping aboard a cruise ship for a little rest and relaxation, you can certainly find options that will keep the scales going in the right direction. Here are a few tips to remember.

Have it your way Whether you're ordering room service or dining at a resort, don't be shy about asking for substitutions: fruit instead of French fries, broccoli instead of fried onion rings, white meat chicken instead of dark meat chicken, wholemeal instead of white bread.

Zero in on healthy options If you're holidaying on an all-inclusive cruise or resort, you will probably be faced with an endless buffet of fattening foods and drinks morning, noon and night – not to mention mid-morning, afternoon and late at night. Use the tips provided earlier on mastering buffets to help you find the best choices amid the dizzying array of calorie bombs.

Keep up with the Quickie Rev Up The Quickie Rev Up has been designed specifically so that you can do it anywhere, anytime. You don't need any equipment, so you can do it in your hotel room, on a sandy beach, or on a cruise ship deck.

Take me out to the match

The Nutrition and Weight Management Center at Boston Medical Center just happens to be located in one of the greatest sports towns in the world. In Boston, people take their sport seriously, and there's nothing better than going to a game. But inside the hallowed halls of Boston's ballparks and arenas lurk some of the most fattening food concoctions you will ever find – and the same is generally true for sports venues in other countries.

Take heart. Going to a game doesn't have to go hand-in-hand with a food binge. In fact, many sports stadiums are adding healthy options to their menus. It's not uncommon to find chicken sandwiches on wholemeal bread, veggie burgers, salads, sushi, raw veggies, fresh produce and fruit. Choose wisely or eat before you go.

At the cinema

For some people, the cinema is where they are most tempted to stray from their new healthy-eating habits. It's easy to see why. As soon as you step into the foyer, your senses are assaulted by the smell of popcorn wafting through the air. But beware of those snacks at the kiosk. They are packed with fat and calories. In fact, a bag of popcorn can have as many calories as a Big Mac, fries and a Coke from McDonald's! This might scare you more than the latest horror flick!

Cinemas have been slow to offer healthy alternatives, but that may be changing. At the 2010 convention of movie theatre owners in the US, it was reported that two-thirds of American moviegoers surveyed would buy healthier concessions if they were available – and there's no reason why cinemagoers else-where should be any different. Until your local cinema is stocked with healthy choices, take your own snacks!

As you can see, it is up to you to take charge of what you con-sume. Don't let a bunch of profit-hungry restaurant, hotel, sports venue and cinema-marketing gurus tell you what to eat. You tell them what you want. Your body will thank you for it.

CHAPTER ELEVEN

....

I Reached My Goal Weight – Now What?

You've made it! After all that time battling with your weight, you're finally seeing that magic number on your scales. Even more exciting, your body isn't just a slimmed-down version of your fatter self, it has been completely re-sculpted, as if someone has chiselled away at it to give your arms, abs, hips, thighs and bottom more definition. Those long, lean muscles you've developed have given you a sleeker figure than you ever imagined. You actually get a kick out of shopping for clothes now because everything fits you better. On top of that, you're bursting with energy. What could be better? Maintaining that toned new shape and vitality for decades to come, that's what.

Losing weight is only half the battle. Keeping it off can be an even tougher challenge. Many people can lose weight – numerous times for some of them – but they haven't found a way to maintain their new smaller size. That's what happened to Claire. She went on a fad crash diet and lost some weight. But when she finished the diet, she went right back to the way she was eating before. It's no surprise Claire quickly ballooned out to her former shape. When Claire went on the Overnight Diet, she wanted to know if it would be any different. Yes, Claire, it is.

The Overnight Diet For Life

Helping you get to your goal weight quickly is only the first part of this diet. Just as much time has been devoted to engineering a post-diet plan to help you maintain that weight loss for the long-term. The Overnight Diet For Life is that plan, and it is designed to maintain the powerful synergy you achieved from this combo diet. By following the Overnight Diet For Life guidelines, you will:

- Maintain your new slimmer waistline.

- Preserve the lean muscle you have developed.

- Keep your metabolism running at lightning-fast speed.

- Keep your fat genes in the 'off' mode.

- Continue to enjoy greater energy.

- Keep water retention and bloating at bay.

- Keep inflammation under control.

- Maintain enhanced insulin sensitivity.

- Minimise your risk of disease.

And the best part is that you can do all this while enjoying an even greater variety of foods.

Tales of the Measuring Tape

'I had lost and regained about 1–2 stone 6 pounds (9.3–13.6kg) at least five times in my lifetime, so I was afraid that I would gain the weight back again this time too. Thank goodness the Overnight Diet comes with a plan on how to keep the weight off once you lose it. I've kept my new weight for three years, and counting!' Sasha, 43, lost 2 stone (13.6kg)

Following the Overnight Diet For Life is easy. Just continue to alternate between the 1-Day Power Up and the 6-Day Fuel Up – with a few very important modification rules.

Rule 1

Modify the 1-Day Power Up to fit your individual needs

The 1-Day Power Up continues to play an important role in maintaining your new physique, but you can modify it depending on your needs and goals. Here are three ways to change your smoothie feast day and still keep the weight off.

Add whole-food snacks Continue to have three jumbo smoothies on the 1-Day Power Up but add two to three small whole-food snacks, such as raw veggies and dip, fruit, cheese wrapped in a slice of turkey or fat-free yogurt. Mariana, 54, who lost 2½ stone (16.3kg) on the diet, has kept it off for almost five years this way. She has a smoothie for breakfast, a piece of fruit, a smoothie for lunch, sliced red pepper and a piece of low-fat cheese, a smoothie for dinner, and then a fat-free yogurt with berries.

Swap one smoothie for a whole meal Switch to having two smoothies a day and one whole meal. It's up to you which meal you prefer – breakfast, lunch or dinner. Thirty-three-year-old Katrina has been following this plan for more than two years since she lost 1 stone 4 pounds (8.2kg) and hasn't gained back a single pound. She likes to whiz up a smoothie for breakfast, eats a full lunch, then sips on another smoothie for dinner. But if she has a business dinner or a night out with friends on her 1-Day Power Up, she simply enjoys smoothies for both breakfast and lunch instead.

Swap two smoothies for whole meals You may find that having just one smoothie along with two solid meals on your 1-Day Power Up will continue to keep you in shape. This combo has been working for 30-year-old Joshua, who shed 1 stone 11 pounds (11.3kg) more than three and a half years ago. He starts his 1-Day Power Up with an invigorating smoothie, then typically has a lunch and a dinner from the 6-Day Fuel Up recipes.

Which option is right for you? After you reach your goal weight, it's best to either include a few whole-food snacks or swap one smoothie for a whole meal. If you continue to lose weight with either of these options, then shift to having two whole-food meals and just one smoothie on your 1-Day Power Up.

Take note that some people find that they really love the way they feel on their smoothie day and want to continue getting the many health benefits a liquid feast day provides. For this reason, they keep following the basic 1-Day Power Up – with three jumbo smoothies a day – long after they have reached their goal weight.

At the age of 46, Lorraine wanted to shed the 1 stone 6 pounds (9.3kg) of excess baggage she had been lugging around since her university days. At first, she was very hesitant to try the 1-Day Power Up and was afraid she would be starving and exhausted all day long. Instead, she found that she felt especially energised on her smoothie day and couldn't be happier that she didn't have to do any cooking on that day. Plus, she loved the idea that she was doing something good for her health. So when Lorraine succeeded in losing that 1 stone 6 pounds (9.3kg), she didn't want to give up her smoothie day. That was almost five years ago, and now aged 51 she is still doing a weekly smoothie day and loving it. She makes sure to eat enough on the other six days of the week to maintain her weight and she feels great.

This is very important: if you ever find yourself gaining a few pounds – say you've overindulged over Christmas or on a holiday – go back to square one. Revert back to the basic 1-Day Power Up to re-ignite fat burning and rapid weight loss, and stick to the basic 6-Day Fuel Up, alternating from one to the other until you get back down to your goal weight.

Rule 2

Tweak the 6-Day Fuel Up for a greater variety of foods

As you progress to the Overnight Diet For Life phase, you will need to make a few modifications to the 6-Day Fuel Up. But that's not a bad thing. You will get to eat an even greater variety of foods that will fill you up and keep you satisfied. I'm talking about including more starchy vegetables like potatoes and sweet potatoes, increasing the number of servings of whole grains you consume, and being a little more generous with those healthy fats. Here's how to tweak the 6-Day Fuel Up.

Keep meeting your DPR every day for life. It is essential that you continue to fuel up on 1.5g of lean protein per kilogram of ideal body weight per day. At this point though, your ideal weight is probably a lot closer to your actual weight. Adequate intake of protein is a big part of what helped you lose the fat and develop lean muscle, and it plays an integral role in allowing you to maintain your new shape. Keep your protein intake at this level throughout the remainder of your life, regardless of your age. As we discussed, getting the right amount and the right kind of protein fuels muscles and boosts metabolism. It also ranks high in terms of satiety, so it keeps you feeling full, which is critical to maintaining weight loss.

Enjoy more starchy vegetables. Love potatoes or parsnips? Feel free to increase your consumption of starchy vegetables to up to around 200g per day. Starchy vegetables include sweetcorn, parsnips, potatoes, sweet potatoes, winter squash, peas, pumpkin and yams. This doesn't mean you can load up your plate with a mound of French fries; that isn't going to help you maintain your weight. But savouring half a baked potato, a serving of peas or sweetcorn, or a few baked sweet potato fries with a meal can satisfy your taste buds and keep your waistline under control. Pay attention to preparation too. Good bets include baking, steaming and boiling.

Eat an extra 1–2 servings of whole grains per day. Bread lovers and pasta lovers, rejoice! I'm giving you permission to eat more of the doughy goodness you love. Just make sure you stick to whole grains rather than refined carbs and watch your portion sizes. One serving means one slice of wholemeal bread, 40–50g of 100 per cent whole-grain cereal, or 80g of cooked brown rice – not one Krispy Kreme doughnut.

Enjoy an extra drizzle of healthy fat. Continue to make healthy PUFAs and MUFAs the main fats in your diet, but feel free to add an extra drizzle, spray or dollop to your meals. This goes for nuts, seeds and avocados too. But don't go crazy dipping your additional servings of wholemeal bread into a bucket of olive oil. Moderation is always essential.

Keep drinking at least 8 glasses of fluids a day and continue savouring a daily glass of wine, if you like. Staying adequately hydrated juices up your metabolism for the long haul. That's why it's important to continue drinking at least eight 250ml glasses of fluids a day. You also get to continue enjoying a nightly glass of wine. Your best bet is to stick with the approved 6-Day Fuel Up fluids for good, because so many fizzy drinks, coffee concoctions, fruit juices, cocktails and energy drinks are loaded with sugar, fat and calories that slow metabolism.

Rule 3

When the Quickie Rev Up starts feeling too easy, ramp up the intensity

When you do the Quickie Rev Up on a regular basis, you will find that moves that seemed really challenging at first start to feel easier. You can do more reps or you can do the reps faster than when you first started. Although you may like the fact that your workout has become easier, your muscles don't. Keeping your muscles challenged is the key to maintaining lean muscle mass. When exercises become too easy for you, switch to the more advanced body-weight moves or try higher-intensity Rev Up Blasts. You'll be ready for it. And if those become too easy, there are many ways to increase the challenge, including using machines at a gym, free weights, kettle bells or medicine balls.

Conclusion – Let Me Help You Keep It Off

In this book, I've given you the guidelines you need to lose 5 pounds (2.25kg), 1 stone (6.3kg) or 3 stone (19kg)-plus and keep it off. I've tried to make this diet as easy as possible to follow, but I know that you may have some questions I didn't anticipate. That's why I have created a website (OvernightDiet.co.uk) where you can go for additional advice, smoothie-making tips and exercise demonstrations (you might even see me demonstrating some of them!), and more. You can also find motivational tips and favourite recipes from other dieters who have already lost the weight or who are on their journey to lasting weight loss just like you. I want to hear from you too, so feel free to share your success, your insights on what's working for you, or your latest sinlessly delicious smoothie creation. With this website, it's like having me as your very own diet doctor guiding you through the weight-loss process so that you can look better, feel better and live longer. Let's do this together.

....

1-Day Power Up Toolkit

Here, you will find helpful tools to create your own 1-Day Power Up smoothies. Discover just some of the amazing flavourings, extracts and spices that can add a powerful punch of taste to your smoothies. And use the step-by-step Mix 'n' Match Smoothie Chart to make your own smoothie creations. You'll find a shopping list that includes ingredients for the 1-Day Power Up in Appendix B.

Mix 'n' Match Smoothie Chart

Protein (choose 1)	1 scoop protein powder, Physicians Protein Mix, whey or soya 250g fat-free Greek yogurt
Liquid (choose 1)	120ml skimmed milk 120ml light soya milk 250ml almond milk, unsweetened 50ml light coconut milk, unsweetened 120ml coconut water 50ml juice of your choice
Fruits (choose up to 2)	½ apple ½ banana 70g cup blueberries 40g cup cherries, pitted

80g cup grapes, seedless
1 kiwi
1 lemon
1 lime
165g mango
1 nectarine, small, pitted
1 orange, small
70g papaya
1 peach
½ pear
80g pineapple
1 plum, pitted
65g raspberries
70g strawberries, sliced

Veggies (choose up to 3)	1 large handful of rocket 1 small carrot 1 celery stalk 50g cucumber, sliced 35g kale, chopped 30g mint leaves 55g Romaine lettuce 35g Swiss chard 30g spinach 1 tomato, small
Add-ins (optional, choose up to 2)	1 tsp agave nectar 1 tbsp avocado 1 tsp blackstrap molasses/black treacle 1 tsp fat-free chocolate syrup 1 tbsp unsweetened cocoa powder 1 tsp smooth peanut butter 1 tbsp rolled oats 1 tsp mixed seeds (flaxseeds, pumpkin, sunflower)

Freebies
(optional, choose
up to 1 of each)
	120ml coffee, brewed
	1 flavouring/extract of your choice, as directed,
	  up to 1 tsp
	120ml green tea, brewed
	¼–½ tsp spice of your choice
	ice – more ice makes smoothie thicker
	salt and freshly ground black pepper, to taste
	1 serving Truvia or Splenda
	water – more water makes the smoothie
	  thinner

Smoothie flavourings and extracts

These food flavourings and extracts are great for adding extra oomph to your smoothies.

Amaretto	Toffee
Anise	Hazelnut
Banana cream	Marshmallow
Butter rum	Peanut butter
Butterscotch	Pecan
Caramel	Peppermint
Champagne	Piña colada
Cheesecake	Pound cake
Coconut	Pralines 'n' cream
Coffee	Pumpkin
Eggnog	

Smoothie herbs and spices

Allspice	Ginger
Anise	Mixed spice
Chilli	Nutmeg
Cinnamon	Orange zest
Cloves	Parsley
Coriander	Wasabi powder

·······················

6-Day Fuel Up Toolkit

To help you prepare for the 6-Day Fuel Up as well as the 1-Day Power Up, use the Overnight Diet shopping list here. This list shows you just how many fruits and vegetables you'll be enjoying on an all-you-can-eat basis. In this Appendix, you'll also discover some cooking tips, a variety of ways to spice up your fruits and veggies for more flavour, and you'll see how some common foods – many of which you'll be consuming on the 6-Day Fuel Up, rate on the Fullness Factor.

The Overnight Diet shopping list

Meat/meat substitutes

☐ Lean beef: thick flank or top rump, topside and silverside, fillet steak

☐ Lean pork: pork chops, pork loin

☐ Fish: cod, haddock, halibut and other white fish; mackerel, salmon, tuna steak and other oily fish; canned tuna/ salmon/sardines in water

☐ Poultry: skinless white meat chicken and turkey

- [ ] Eggs
- [ ] Tofu, tempeh or other soya products

Protein powders

- [ ] Soya protein isolate
- [ ] Whey protein isolate
- [ ] Physicians Protein Mix

Milk and milk products

- [ ] Milk, skimmed or semi-skimmed
- [ ] Dairy alternatives, fat-free or low-fat, unsweetened
- [ ] Cottage cheese, low-fat
- [ ] Cheese, low-fat
- [ ] Greek yogurt, fat-free, no fruit added
- [ ] Dessert, fat-free, sugar-free

Fruit (all-you-can-eat)

- [ ] Apples
- [ ] Avocados
- [ ] Bananas
- [ ] Blackberries
- [ ] Blueberries
- [ ] Cherries
- [ ] Clementines
- [ ] Figs
- [ ] Grapefruit
- [ ] Grapes
- [ ] Guava
- [ ] Kiwi
- [ ] Lemons
- [ ] Limes
- [ ] Mangoes

- [ ] Melons
- [ ] Nectarines
- [ ] Oranges
- [ ] Papayas
- [ ] Peaches
- [ ] Pears
- [ ] Pineapple
- [ ] Plums
- [ ] Pomegranates
- [ ] Raspberries
- [ ] Star fruit
- [ ] Strawberries
- [ ] Fruit canned in water or own juice, not syrup

Non-starchy vegetables (all-you-can-eat)

- [ ] Artichokes
- [ ] Asparagus
- [ ] Aubergine
- [ ] Bamboo shoots
- [ ] Beans
- [ ] Bean sprouts
- [ ] Beetroot
- [ ] Broccoli
- [ ] Brussels sprouts
- [ ] Cabbage
- [ ] Carrots
- [ ] Cauliflower
- [ ] Celery
- [ ] Courgettes
- [ ] Cucumbers
- [ ] Greens (spring greens, Swiss chard)
- [ ] Kale

- [ ] Kohlrabi
- [ ] Leeks
- [ ] Lettuce
- [ ] Mushrooms
- [ ] Mange tout
- [ ] Okra
- [ ] Onions
- [ ] Peppers
- [ ] Sauerkraut
- [ ] Spinach
- [ ] Spring onions
- [ ] Sprouts (alfalfa, mung bean, lentil)
- [ ] Swede
- [ ] Tomatoes
- [ ] Turnips
- [ ] Water chestnuts

Starchy vegetables/pulses

- [ ] Black beans
- [ ] Black-eyed beans
- [ ] Butter beans
- [ ] Cannellini beans
- [ ] Chickpeas
- [ ] Haricot beans
- [ ] Kidney beans
- [ ] Lentils
- [ ] Peas
- [ ] Pinto beans
- [ ] Potatoes
- [ ] Pumpkin and squash
- [ ] Split peas
- [ ] Sweet potatoes

- [ ] Sweetcorn
- [ ] Yams

Whole grains

- [ ] Bagel, wholemeal
- [ ] Bread, wholemeal
- [ ] Couscous
- [ ] Oatmeal
- [ ] Pasta, whole-wheat
- [ ] Quinoa
- [ ] Rice, brown basmati
- [ ] Crackers, wholegrain or rye

Fats & fat alternatives

- [ ] Almonds
- [ ] Cashew nuts
- [ ] Cooking spray, made from olive oil
- [ ] Cumin seeds
- [ ] Fennel seeds
- [ ] Flaxseeds
- [ ] Flaxseed oil
- [ ] Mayonnaise, fat-free or low-fat
- [ ] Olive oil
- [ ] Peanuts
- [ ] Peanut butter
- [ ] Pine nuts
- [ ] Pumpkin seeds
- [ ] Salad dressings, fat-free or low-fat
- [ ] Sesame seeds
- [ ] Sunflower seeds
- [ ] Walnuts

Sweets
- [ ] Artificial sweeteners (Truvia, Splenda)
- [ ] Chocolate chips
- [ ] Chocolate syrup, fat-free
- [ ] Cocoa powder, unsweetened
- [ ] Dried fruits
- [ ] Sugar-free jelly
- [ ] Sugar-free chewing gum

Condiments
- [ ] Basil
- [ ] Celery powder
- [ ] Garlic powder
- [ ] Lemon juice
- [ ] Lime juice
- [ ] Mustard
- [ ] Onion powder
- [ ] Oregano
- [ ] Pepper
- [ ] Salt
- [ ] Spices, flavourings, extracts
- [ ] Vinegar

Beverages
- [ ] Cocoa powder, fat-free, unsweetened
- [ ] Coffee
- [ ] Flavoured water
- [ ] Juice (for smoothies only)
- [ ] Tea
- [ ] Tomato juice
- [ ] Water

Spice up your veggies

Which herbs, spices and condiments go best with which vegetables? Use this handy chart to find combinations you love.

Asparagus	Garlic, lemon juice, mustard, onion, paprika, parsley, tarragon, vinegar
Aubergine	Marjoram, oregano
Broccoli	Caraway seed, curry, dill, garlic, mustard, tarragon
Brussels sprouts	Basil, caraway, dill, garlic, mustard, sage, thyme
Cabbage	Caraway, celery seed, dill, mint, mustard, nutmeg, tarragon
Carrots	Allspice, bay leaves, caraway, curry, dill, ginger, mace, marjoram, mint, nutmeg, parsley, thyme
Cauliflower	Caraway, curry, dill, garlic, mace, paprika, saffron, tarragon
Cucumber	Basil, chives, dill, garlic, mint, parsley, tarragon, vinegar
Courgettes	Basil, fresh coriander, garlic, oregano, paprika, parsley, saffron, tarragon
Green beans	Basil, dill, garlic, lemon juice, marjoram, mint, mustard, nutmeg, oregano, paprika, parsley, tarragon, thyme
Green salads	Basil, chives, dill, parsley, tarragon
Mushrooms	Garlic, oregano, paprika, pepper, saffron, sage
Onions	Caraway, chilli, fresh coriander, curry, garlic, mustard, nutmeg, oregano, paprika, saffron, sage, thyme
Pumpkin and squash	Garlic, oregano, paprika, saffron, tarragon, basil
Spinach	Basil, garlic, mace, marjoram, nutmeg, oregano, saffron
Tomatoes	Basil, bay leaves, celery, chilli, fresh coriander, garlic, marjoram, oregano, parsley, sage, tarragon, thyme

Spice up your fruit

Herbs and spices that enhance the flavour of fruit.

Cinnamon

Cloves

Coriander

Mint leaves

Peppermint

Poppy seeds

Spearmint

Vanilla

Fruits and vegetables high in antioxidants

Acai berries

Avocados

Beetroot

Blackberries

Blueberries

Broccoli

Brussels sprouts

Carrots

Cherries

Cranberries

Kale

Kiwi fruit

Oranges

Plums

Pomegranates

Raspberries

Red peppers

Red grapes

Spinach

Strawberries

Index